ALL ABOUT
ME

LOVING A NARCISSIST

SIMON
CROMPTON

Collins

First published in 2007 by Collins,

an imprint of HarperCollins Publishers Ltd.
77–85 Fulham Palace Road
London
W6 8JB

www.collins.co.uk

8 7 6 5 4 3 2 1
11 10 09 08 07

A catalogue record for this book is
available from the British Library.

ISBN-10: 0-00-724795-8
ISBN-13: 978-0-00-724795-0

Set by Rowland Phototypesetting Ltd, Bury St Edmunds, Suffolk

Printed and bound in Great Britain by Clays Ltd, St Ives plc

This book is proudly printed on paper which contains wood
from well managed forests, certified in accordance with
the rules of the Forest Stewardship Council.
For more information about FSC,
please visit www.fsc-uk.org

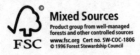

Mixed Sources
Product group from well-managed
forests and other controlled sources
www.fsc.org Cert no. SW-COC-1806
© 1996 Forest Stewardship Council

CONTENTS

INTRODUCTION

Why do women fall in love with bad guys? It's a question that worried me and countless other males in their tender years when we never seemed to get the girl. It was always the mean, arrogant ones who seemed to succeed.

Why was it, I asked myself as I struggled to make an impression in my twenties, that the same self-centred show-offs who got the girls were now also getting the top jobs and glamorous lifestyles? They seemed to be rising to the top like cream (or fat, depending on your perspective). Whatever happened to the benefits of trying to be a nice guy?

Not that I was bitter. But then, as the years rolled on, I saw my arguably warped perspective changing, and what emerged was not pretty. I saw the relationships involving moody self-glorifiers proving far from idyllic and beginning to break up. I saw those grandiose schemes and high-flying lifestyles begin to crumble. And there seemed to be an awful lot of collateral damage and emotional debris left in these people's wake.

This, in a sense, is what this book is about. It's about a type of human personality – glamorous, self-centred, difficult, and intensely vulnerable – that we call narcissistic. Narcissists are people who are full of big ideas of themselves and for themselves, but they need others to reflect their glory, and find real empathy almost impossible. They are people who mean trouble when it comes to relationships.

There are a lot of them around, and you're bound to have come across them. In fact, if you've picked up this book, you're probably wondering whether your partner is a narcissist or not. It's a good question, and the answer is probably yes – although, as we'll see, there's a world of a difference between someone who shows narcissistic traits, which is far from uncommon, and someone who is a full-blown narcissistic personality.

This book is about the hold narcissists have on us – how they are easy to fall in love with, how they have a major influence on our culture, how they can damage the lives of those around them, and how they can be incredibly hard to disentangle yourself from.

But it's also a book about all of us. Narcissism is a concept, not a diagnosis. In other words, it describes common characteristics in human beings. We all need a bit of narcissism – a bit of self-centredness, a bit of overwhelming self-regard – to be able do anything, to feel good about ourselves, to impose ourselves a little. It's just that in some people, those tendencies can be consistently dominant, even overwhelming, and that means trouble.

Ever spent much time with a toddler? Then you'll have experienced narcissism. For all their allure, babies and toddlers are unable to see the world from anyone else's perspective apart from their own. Don't get what you want? Then throw your rattle out of the pram. It's quite natural and programmed into them – into all human beings. But as we get older, through the influence of our parents and others, most of us lose that self-regarding, impulsive streak to a greater or lesser extent – we learn that there are consequences to our actions, and that we have to take into account the needs and wants of others if we are to be happy.

Throughout history, some of us have never learned those lessons, and continue to act like toddlers. It's part of human life, achievement and tragedy, and it influences every one of us. It's narcissism, and it makes us the flawed and fascinating things we are.

Once you begin to understand narcissism – and to use it as a lens through which to see much of human behaviour – then lots of things that are mystifying and frustrating about people, relationships and our culture begin to fall into place. Relationships in particular.

Take this plea for help in an online agony column:

♥

Hi. This may seem silly but it hurts me. The thing is, my friends invite me and my boyfriend out every time they are going out, and when I ask my boyfriend if he wants to go out he always makes up an excuse. Like on Saturday, my friends had arranged to go for a night out and asked me and my boyfriend to go, and when I asked him he said maybe. Then two hours later he said he wasn't feeling well. But then his sister phoned and asked if we wanted to go and play pool and he said yeah. We got into an argument because I thought he was being selfish, because my friends had asked first. When I asked if he had a problem with my friends, he said no, he just didn't want to go. We ended up staying in that night but he hardly spoke to me. I asked him the following morning why he had hardly spoken to me the night before. He said that it was because he wanted to go play pool. Is he being selfish, or am I just being silly?

♥

As the writer says, this sounds like old-fashioned selfishness. But it can also be explained by her boyfriend showing narcissism – a particular form of selfishness that targets people with either lavish attention or hostility, that makes loved ones isolated, and that blames others for personal shortcomings. As you'll see further on in the book, this can have far more disastrous effects on relationships than arguments about not seeing friends.

I was talking to the journalist, novelist and relationships writer Bel Mooney about this. The idea of narcissism, she said, helped explain many of the letters she got from readers writing in to her regular advice column in *The Times*. In recent years, she said, she's noted an increase in people writing to her who are, to use an old-fashioned phrase, 'self-centred'.

'It's all I, I, I, I, I,' she said. 'They go on about themselves in a very self-indulgent way, talking about how they need to find themselves and so on. And I think, "Why are you asking me what to do, because what you really want me to do is to confirm what you are feeling, and if I challenge it you aren't going to like it." And I think, how are those people going to be in a relationship? And I'd say dire.

'You get letters from these sorts of people wishing that others could be satellites around their sun. I've been amazed at the number of stories like that I've had since I started the column – people who are so lacking in empathy that you feel something is very missing. The problem is serious because at its more extreme end it can go into personality disorder.'

She told me of one letter from a man whose 40-year-old wife had become increasingly obsessive about her appearance and weight, constantly going to the gym. He discovered she was having a relationship with another man at the gym because of the texts she had been sending him, and when he confronted her with this she became violent and abusive with him in front of the children. She became increasingly critical of him, and then asked for a separation. 'I don't know whether that's narcissism or not, but it is common and extremely cruel,' Bel told me.

Well, yes, it is narcissism, and it does manifest itself in very cruel ways in relationships. But as we'll see in the rest of this book, the concept of narcissism also throws light on all sorts of other aspects of our lives: it makes sense of our ideas of romantic heroes, of obsessively driven high-achievers, of compulsive liars and doomed and deluded dreamers. It makes sense of our glamour-led, celebrity-obsessed culture. It makes sense of our society's obsession with high-achievement and winning at all costs. It even makes sense of our *Truman Show*-style love affair with reality television, and all those *X Factor* contenders who believe against all the evidence that they really will be the next Christina Aguilera or Justin Timberlake.

Think of those high-profile politicians whose relationship with the truth has been, shall we say, tenuous. Richard Nixon, Bill Clinton, Jeffrey Archer ... all have been caught lying in a big way. Their behaviour can be explained in the context of the narcissistic traits that made them big achievers in the first place. With their vision and drive for success came a tendency to the fantastical that is classic narcissism, and makes lying less of a sin and more of an inner compulsion.

Narcissistic personalities are, and always have been, intrinsic to human attraction, achievement and tragedy. But today, in the navel-gazing, celebrity-exposing noughties, they are more apparent than ever before. If there ever were one, this is the Age of the Narcissist.

♥

In the therapy-obsessed United States, narcissism is a household word. It is used to explain sundry acts of cruelty, selfishness and grandiosity among the population. The internet message-boards of Dr Phil, America's top agony uncle, are full of people suddenly realising that their problems are the result of having narcissistic parents.

Why have the Americans latched onto this term in such a big

way? It probably all started with a hugely popular book written by sociologist Christopher Lasch in 1979 called *The Culture of Narcissism*. It was an indictment of the increasingly self-centred short-termism of American society, as sense of family and society declined. It drove the word 'narcissism' firmly into popular American usage. Not long after came the classification of a new personality disorder by the American Psychiatric Association – it was called Narcissistic Personality Disorder. After that came a personal mission by self-confessed narcissist and author Sam Vaknin to raise the profile of the condition, through a book and continued high profile on the internet.

Since then, the diagnosis and treatment of the disorder has spawned a string of books, been the subject of hundreds of chat shows, and given rise to dozens of support groups and online chat forums where victims of narcissists share their stories of suffering at the hands of manipulative men and women.

The focus over the Atlantic is very much on narcissism as a dangerous disorder – a psychiatric problem. 'Narcissists lack empathy, are exploitative, envious, haughty and feel entitled, even if such a feeling is commensurate only with their grandiose fantasies,' writes Sam Vaknin. 'They dissemble, conspire, destroy and self-destruct. In the long run, there is no enduring benefit to dancing with narcissists – only ephemeral and, often, fallacious "achievements".'[1]

Not nice people then. Over here, the popular view is a bit different. When most of us hear the word 'narcissist', we don't tend to think of people with a personality disorder. We still tend to think of a narcissistic man as a preening Brad Pitt type, who hones his abs and pecs, occasionally plucks his eyebrows and assesses his own reflection when he looks into your eyes. It's people like David Beckham who get called narcissists in Britain, because they care about their looks and have a standing and image that they do their damnedest to maintain.[2] Because the British are naturally suspicious of anyone who cares too much about what others think of them, the term here is still mainly reserved as a vague form of mild abuse. We are far less aware of the specific meaning of the word in psychoanalytic or psychiatric terms.

But things are beginning to change. In July 2005 the film star Jude Law, dubbed the world's sexiest man by *People* magazine, admitted an affair with a family nanny. Reports followed, supposedly from a 'source close to Ms Miller' that actress Sienna Miller, his partner, had as a result given Law an ultimatum: he must make her fall in love with him all over again, he must control his temper, he must not stop her from seeing her friends.

The reports gave way to media speculation that Jude Law did, in fact, show all the traits of a narcissist. 'It's the musts that give it away,' wrote Yvonne Roberts in the *Independent*, 'as does the graphic picture presented in the press of a controlling, possessive, cheating individual who doesn't appear to know what he wants until it's in danger of slipping away.'[3] These, she explained, were some of the traits associated with a condition called narcissistic personality disorder, widely diagnosed in the

United States. 'In the Sixties, the common slogan was "All men are bastards". Now for those in the know, fairly or unfairly, it's "All men are narcissistic bastards".'

Who knows if Jude Law really is a narcissist? But I like the new slogan, because narcissism does (as we'll see later in the book) indeed help explain why men are bastards.

What is interesting is the way the story exemplifies the new importance of narcissism in our culture, and the way we view relationships. The characters Jude Law plays in his films sometimes exemplify the traits of narcissism – look at Alfie in the film of the same name, for example: remote, self-regarding, womanising and incapable of empathy. These are the kind of anti-heroes that have gained increasing currency as leading men in film and television culture. There's something about them that draws and keeps our attention. Those same qualities seem to have rubbed off on the actor in real life, drawing a feverish interest from the media and among the public. We watch the every move of the glamorous and famous because we aspire to look like them and be like them. So the appeal of narcissism draws out our own narcissistic tendencies.

Yet beneath it all, if you look at Jude Law and his family, there's a real story of pain. We don't know what happened in his household, and it would be unfair to label Law a narcissist on hearsay. But we do know that people with strong narcissistic traits tend not to be happy people, and find family life hard. Having a relationship with a narcissist is a rollercoaster where the lows can drag all sense of self-worth out of the partner.

So what I hope to show in this book is that narcissism is a far deeper and far more useful idea than the British have previously given it credit for. And it's a far broader, less medicalised idea than the Americans have given it credit for. As a health and relationships writer, I come to the subject with a very broad perspective. You'll find other books on narcissism (if you search hard enough) that look at it from a psychoanalytical point of view, or from a relationships counselling point of view, or a cultural point of view. What I want to do with this book is take a wider approach, combining the above with the medical, the evolutionary, the psychiatric, the sociological and the historical. This is not a specialist or an academic book on narcissism – it is a book to help us try to understand our relationships with people and the world. Because if this is indeed the Age of Narcissism, we need to understand how the concept is shaping our world and relationships in all its different ways.

There are dangers in addressing a subject like this. As a journalist, I'm very aware of how easy it is to label people for the sake of convenience. There's an increasing tendency among popular psychoanalysis and psychology to force human nature into boxes neatly labelled 'personality type'. There's another, and linked, tendency for doctors, psychiatrists and drug manufacturers to try to turn personality traits into illnesses. Once we were just a 'type', now we have a diagnosis. There are lots of examples. Many thousands of children are now being diagnosed with ADHD (attention deficit hyperactivity disorder), which was unheard of 30 years ago. Some people are controversially saying that the condition doesn't really exist. It's simply what a few decades ago would have been classified as 'wilfully naughty children', they say. The children haven't changed, but our attitude to them has.

There is a similar controversy raging over autistic spectrum disorders – some are claiming that many of these conditions, such as Asperger's Syndrome, are not disorders at all – merely different manifestations of 'maleness'.

These are difficult areas. But whatever you believe about ADHD and autism, it's certainly true that a large number of drug companies are now trialling drugs designed specifically to combat all sorts of behavioural traits that until recently most of us would simply have regarded as all being on the continuum of 'normal': stress, shyness, anxiety, phobias, gambling, impulsive behaviours – even addiction to the internet.

I don't want to do the same kind of thing for narcissism or suggest that something which up to now has been regarded as a human trait of selfishness should become a formal tag to put onto people willy-nilly. But seeing patterns in relationships and the way we conduct our lives helps us to overcome problems, and talking about narcissism can help us understand some of the people in our lives and some of the pitfalls in our own behaviour that can make us more vulnerable to them. It helps us to identify when we are the victims of narcissism, and ways we can assist each other to break out of destructive, self-centred cycles. It also helps identify the small number of people who need expert psychiatric help because they have a genuine personality disorder.

So forgive me if I use the tags 'narcissist' or 'narcissistic personality' in the following chapters. I'm not suggesting that the people being referred to are only narcissists, or that they don't have many other characteristics too. Humans are an intricate bundle of motivations and behaviours. But I hope to make it clear that in some people, narcissistic traits are sufficiently character-defining for us to have justification in calling them narcissists.

You'll see in the next chapter that the word has a long history of describing human characteristics, from Greek myth, via Freud, into modern psychiatric textbooks and popular usage. That makes it different and arguably richer than other, simpler human personality traits such as, say, 'anger' or 'selfishness'. What's more, there's an increasing consensus that the causes of narcissism lie in the way we are brought up. It raises fascinating questions about parenting, and the interaction between our genetic make-up and our environment in conditioning our personality.

The book also deals with how narcissism has affected relationships, how different individuals have coped, and some of the coping strategies you can try to implement if narcissism is having a negative effect on your life. You'll read in the chapters 'I'm a celebrity narcissist' and 'Generation me' about the dangers we all face as we are unwittingly drawn into a cult of narcissism, where the selfish and self-obsessed values that create narcissists are also being promoted as desirable and glamorous in our popular culture.

I started out writing a book because I was intrigued about
the men who seemed to succeed at everything, and I ended up
writing a book not just about them, but about all of us. About
the vulnerability that can make us behave in strange and difficult
ways, and which leaves us susceptible to the charms of those
who will make life most troublesome for us. Like the tale of
Narcissus itself, it's a very human story. Anyone who has ever
felt used by the one they love, anyone who feels that others have
needed them merely to prop up their ego, and anyone who has
ever been humiliated in a relationship should read on . . .

Notes

[1] Sam Vaknin was writing on Amazon's pages, reviewing Michael
   Maccoby's book *The Productive Narcissist*.

[2] Jeff Powell, 'Good riddance to the game's golden fleecer', *Daily
   Mail*, 3 July 2006.

[3] Yvonne Roberts, '"I want" is the slogan of our age', *Independent*,
   22 September 2005.

1

IT'S ALL ABOUT ME

What is a narcissist?

Enough about me.
We've talked far too much about me,
let's talk about you.
What do you think about me?

So you want to know what a narcissist is? It's all those annoying people who are more conscious of image than substance, isn't it? Those hollow gym bunnies, those self-centred people who are so interested in how fabulous they are that they can't even see how glorious you happen to be looking this evening? Possibly even someone like your boyfriend, or girlfriend?

Well, that's certainly part of the story. *Narcissism* is a word that's increasingly bandied around by the media as a means of describing intensely self-centred or image-conscious people.

If you saw politician George Galloway's preening, arrogant performance on Channel 4's *Celebrity Big Brother* in 2006, it will come as no surprise that David Aaronovitch commented in *The Times* that 'it was the narcissist, not the politician, who had turned up to compete'.[1]

Welsh rugby player Gavin Henson is another modern-day narcissist by popular definition. He was 'outed' by girlfriend Charlotte Church in July 2006 as having an extensive beauty regime, including constantly changing the side he sleeps on to avoid getting lines on his face. He's reported as saying it takes him two hours to get ready before a rugby game. 'Hot bath, shave my legs and face, moisturise, put fake tan on and do my hair. I need my fellow players to say I'm looking good.'[2]

You'll have heard the term 'narcissist' being commonly bandied around as an alternative to the tag of 'metrosexual', applied to image-conscious celebs like David Beckham, Thierry Henry and even Tony Blair.[3] This everyday use is all about image, self-obsession and vanity. Narcissists are just people who love themselves, aren't they?

Well, not just that. There's a far more specific meaning of the word *narcissist*, revolving around the way we live our lives and conduct our relationships. It has been used by generations of psychoanalysts to describe a specific form of human behaviour.

Here's what a woman called Mandy thinks a narcissist is. She finished with her boyfriend after a two-year relationship. Then, on the internet, she saw accounts from other women who believed their relationships had foundered because their partners had 'narcissistic personalities' – not simply vain, but so self-centred that they were incapable of giving love and were only using their partner as a means to inflate their own ego. It rang so many bells for Mandy that it made her view her past relationship in a new light of understanding. This is what she says:

♥

I really thought that I loved him. I thought that telling him I loved him and that I'd never leave him would somehow ease what I perceived to be his fear of abandonment. I put up with him never being loving and I believed him when he said that yelling at me was his way of showing me how much he loved me. He called it passion. When he was with other people, he was completely different. Everyone who met him said he was always singing my praises, saying how much he loved me.

Even now we've finished, he's always in touch, promoting all the great things he's done, and saying how fantastic he is. But now I get some satisfaction in knowing that he's a narcissist – an empty shell who must constantly feed off others – and I'm well out of it. He isn't capable of love. He's a terrified chameleon who takes on the persona that will best please the person who's feeding his ego at that particular moment.

♥

It's a powerful portrait, and illustrates the point that narcissism goes far beyond strutting like a peacock. Narcissistic people have a sense of self-importance that depends on the admiration of others – and often ends up damaging others because of the narcissist's inability to understand how they feel. Their innate uncertainty about their own worth gives rise to them concocting a self-protective, but often totally spurious, aura of grandiosity. It may not always be as extreme as in Mandy's description, but it is common.

This more worrying definition is very closely linked to the popular idea of narcissists as self-obsessed clothes horses. Here, at the beginning of the twenty-first century, a new and multi-faceted understanding of the word is emerging, combining elements of previous interpretations down the decades. As the centuries have passed, new levels of meaning have stuck like barnacles to what originated as Greek myth. And as the idea of narcissism has gained increasing complexity, it also describes something very fundamental about human nature and the relationships we have with each other and our world. It is a concept that allows us to identify and characterise some of the defining aspects of personality.

WHAT ANCIENT MYTH TELLS US ABOUT NARCISSISM

You can't talk about narcissism without telling the story of Narcissus, the beautiful son of a minor Greek god. The story is found (appropriately enough for a concept that has undergone regular transformation over the decades) in a collection of stories called *Metamorphoses* by the Roman poet Ovid. It's the story of a boy who can't stop staring at his reflection in a pond, while the woman who loves him pines away, ignored.

That in itself tells us a lot about the modern meaning of narcissism. It's not just about vanity, but about the terrible human consequences for yourself and those around you if you are so transfixed by yourself that you are unable to understand the feelings of others, or engage with them.

The details of the story give rise to other fundamental notions of narcissism. It's about glamour, isolation and terrible unspoken suffering. Self-absorption is at the very root of its tragedy.

Narcissus, the 16-year-old son of the river god Cephissus, is so beautiful that all the nymphs in the woods where he hunts fall in love with him. But he rejects them all. One of the nymphs, Echo, becomes so distraught over his indifference that she withdraws to a lonely spot and, as she fades away in her grief, she prays that one day Narcissus might feel for himself what it is like to love and not have that love returned.

The avenging goddess Nemesis hears Echo's words, and grants her wishes.

Soon after, while Narcissus is out hunting, he comes to a clear fountain that he has never seen before, and bends down to drink. In the water, he sees his own reflection – and thinking that the image belongs to some beautiful spirit living in the pool, he gazes at the face adoringly. He doesn't know it, but he has fallen in love with his own reflection.

When he tries to kiss the spirit, it disappears in the ripples. It vanishes when he tries to hold it, thrusting his hands into the water. But, almost instantly, it returns as the water smoothes, renewing his fascination and tantalising him once again.

Narcissus cannot tear himself away from the water, or stop looking into it, and he is so infatuated that he loses all thought of food or drink. But the more he longs, the more he cries. And as his tears fall in the water, they send the beautiful face away again, making him even more inconsolable. As the poet Ted Hughes wrote, in his translation of *Ovid*: 'He was himself/ The torturer who now began his torture.'[4]

Like Echo, Narcissus loses his vigour and beauty. He pines away and dies. But when the mourning nymphs come to collect his body to put it on the funeral pyre, they cannot find it. In its place, at the spot where he died, there is only a beautiful white flower.

WHAT PSYCHOANALYSTS TELL US ABOUT NARCISSISM

The first person to take the myth of Narcissus and give it a specific significance in describing human nature was the British doctor, sexual psychologist and social reformer Havelock Ellis in 1898. He used it to describe a form of pathological self-absorption. But it was the father of psychoanalysis, Sigmund Freud, who in the early twentieth century tied the idea of Narcissus more specifically to human psychological traits, and presented the first coherent theory of narcissism in human beings.

Freud said that narcissism was a natural part of the human makeup, but also a characteristic that if taken to extremes can prevent us from having meaningful relationships. In 1914, Freud distinguished between primary narcissism and secondary narcissism. Primary narcissism, he said, is the love of self in our infancy which precedes our ability to love others. It is a natural and essential stage of the child's development, when a child asserts a sense of identity – learning how to love themselves before they can love anyone else.[5] This idea of the formation of the 'self' in childhood has been built on by many of Freud's followers in psychoanalysis. The French psychoanalyst and philosopher Jacques Lacan, for example, put a new twist on primary narcissism by developing a theory of the 'mirror phase', where babies develop a sense of self and others only once they have recognised their own reflection in a mirror.

Secondary narcissism is something very different – a form of self-love that people can develop in adulthood when they should be well beyond primary narcissism and should have learned to find external objects for their love. Secondary narcissism is a form of regression back to childish self-absorption, as a result of having tried to reach out to objects of desire, but failing to gain their love or attention. It is, in effect, a means of protecting yourself against further rejection.

These ideas are still relevant to modern and emerging ideas of narcissism. When we talk about narcissists today, we are referring to secondary narcissists – people who are stuck in, or reverting to, childish self-centredness. Freud's work demonstrates that 'narcissist' isn't just an abusive term – it's something inherent in all of us, and something that we are all liable to fall back on as a result of emotional trauma.

Freud's definitions are important because they set the groundwork for our increasing understanding that people become narcissistic and self-regarding not because they are simply 'bad' or 'difficult' but because they are vulnerable. There's now a widely-held belief that real narcissism in adulthood usually has its roots in emotional rejection or deprivation from one's parents in childhood. It's a pattern born of a lack of empathy and love, and results in people being in turn unable to empathise or love. Narcissists breed narcissists, because their behaviour forces their children to create an artificial idea of grandiosity and self-esteem around themselves. It's self-defence.

Many psychoanalysts have pointed out that it's not just our relationships with our parents that can encourage narcissistic tendencies – it's our relationship with other people and society too. Freud's followers have picked up on the term 'narcissism', because it seems increasingly relevant to our modern times.

As psychoanalyst Marion F Solomon says, many people today suffer from 'a narcissistic vulnerability that permeates all their relationships'. This is the result, she says, of a number of converging factors, including 'the messages that society sends us, the emotional failure between parents and children, and the history of failed relationships that has today become part of the life of many.' Narcissistically vulnerable people desperately wish to be involved in a relationship, but have unreasonable expectations of what they should give to the relationship, and what they should get from it. This inevitably leads to disappointment and frustration for both themselves and their partners.[6]

Because of our experiences, some of us have strong narcissistic traits in adulthood, and others have milder ones. All of us will have narcissistic traits as children. And all of us are likely to revert to narcissistic, self-centred patterns of behaviour at times of stress. We all become needy and demanding when we feel we can't cope. This has a name: it's called reactive narcissistic regression. Even if you're the most empathetic, selfless person around, you'll have some understanding of narcissism if you try to imagine how it feels when you've been really upset and are demanding attention. Say you've just had an argument with someone you love. You'll cry and make a scene and make demands on people – probably your friends – that you would never do normally. You might even exaggerate your own achievements a bit to boost your own sense of power, and compensate for the vulnerability you are feeling inside. 'I told him like it was ... I'm too good for him, and he knows it.' That's you, essentially, reverting to a primary narcissistic state. The thing about people with strong narcissistic traits is that they are like that most of the time.

WHY NARCISSISM IS GETTING SERIOUS

In the 1970s, two psychoanalysts from America – Heinz Kohut and Otto Kernberg – played a major part in defining modern ideas of narcissism. Though they disagreed on the causes, they put forward ideas of narcissism as a 'disorder of the personality' that has been widely taken up in popular American culture. Kohut was the man who first coined the phrase 'narcissistic personality disorder', saying that some of the traits that Freud and other psychoanalysts had classified as narcissistic could be so problematic in some people that they constituted a personality disorder.[7]

This had a real impact, particularly after 1980, when narcissistic personality disorder, or NPD, was recognised as a distinct mental health disorder by the American Psychiatric Association. Examples of personality disorders in the same category as narcissistic personality disorder include antisocial personality disorder and borderline personality disorder.

Suddenly, narcissism had distinct 'diagnostic criteria', and NPD was a clinical term that could be legitimately used of people who have 'an excessive sense of how important they are', and who 'demand and expect to be admired and praised by others and are limited in their capacity to appreciate others' perspectives'.[8]

This is a controversial area. Not everyone, including some psychiatric authorities in the UK, is convinced that moving psychoanalytical theories about personality types and the evolution of a sense of self into the arena of diagnosable mental-health problems is helpful – particularly when the treatment for that particular illness is unknown. Their fears are perhaps supported by what has happened in the United States since word about NPD hit the agony aunts, the chat shows and the pages of dozens of books.

Therapy-literate Americans are now rushing to diagnose others, and themselves, as narcissistic personalities – not in a 'It's natural for us all to have narcissistic tendencies but some are more narcissistic than others' kind of way, but in a 'narcissism is bad' kind of way, involving much pointing of accusatory fingers. The word 'toxic' is now regularly attached to the word 'narcissism', and millions of American men and women are taking the diagnostic criteria for NPD, overlaying them onto their foundering relationships, and condemning their partners as narcissistic personalities.

There's much breast-beating too. Bestselling relationship authors Steven Carter and Julia Sokol, who wrote the book *Help! I'm in Love with a Narcissist!*, confess that when they started to research their book, they began to see aspects of themselves in many of the case histories and behaviour patterns they were writing about. 'It is a terrible thing to be writing a book about "awful behaviors" and "awful people" only to realise that you share some of their characteristics' they wrote.

Perhaps they should take stock of their own wise advice later in their book, where they point out that most of us have some narcissistic or selfish characteristics. 'That doesn't make us awful or completely unpleasant to know. It does make us human, with room for improvement.'[9]

Because the truth is that narcissistic personality disorder and narcissism are closely related, but not the same thing. They are different points on a continuum of human characteristics – just as obsessive attention to detail and genuine autism are points at different ends of a spectrum of human characteristics. So narcissism may be difficult, 'toxic' and even dangerous in some people, but it's important to see it in a wider perspective. If only because, if it's in all of us to some extent, we cannot use it too readily as a weapon to hurl at others. The key is understanding. As the British psychoanalyst Michael Knight said when I spoke to him: 'All of us have personality disorders on a bad day.'

That's not to say that the American Psychological Association's definition isn't useful – it is, not least in pinning down some of the most commonly observed traits of the people we have come to describe as narcissists. The American Psychological Association's diagnostic definition of NPD is carefully put together, and tells us a lot about narcissists at all points on the continuum – their exaggerated sense of self-importance and fantasies of their brilliance and success, for example. It tells us that they believe they are special, and that they are entitled to admiration or favourable treatment. It tells us that they tend to take advantage of others to achieve their ends, and find it hard to identify with the feelings of others. And it tells us that narcissists are often arrogant and haughty.

People who have several of those characteristics, manifesting themselves in such a consistent and extreme manner that they severely disrupt lives, may well be described as having a personality disorder. Those who sometimes show signs of some of them are simply displaying narcissistic traits. The extent to which they need addressing depends on how problematic they are proving – either for the individual concerned, or for the person they are having a relationship with. The fact that they do indeed often prove problematic, particularly for the people whose lives they touch, is one of the main reasons why narcissism demands our attention.

SAM VAKNIN AND THE CULT OF NARCISSISM

Sam who? Sam Vaknin is one of the most influential voices in modern perceptions of narcissism. This is partly because of his book, *Malignant Self Love – Narcissism Revisited*. But mainly it is because of his amazingly intense presence on the internet – in discussion forums, information pages, agony columns. He is not a psychoanalyst or a psychologist or a psychotherapist. In fact he's a philosopher. But he's also a self-confessed narcissist, and has become a self-appointed spokesman on narcissism issues for America – and, via the internet, the world.

Vaknin doesn't go easy on narcissistic personalities. He regularly comments on their 'toxicity' or 'malignancy'. A typical comment on narcissists is: 'The glamour and trickery wear thin and underneath them a monster lurks which irreversibly and adversely influences the lives of those around it for the worse.'

Vaknin has his detractors. Some people have criticised him for recreating narcissism in his own image – appropriately enough.[10] Others believe he satisfies his own narcissistic needs by creating himself as a guru to whom women (mainly) in distress turn to for advice. But his considerable industry on the subject has had a major effect on making narcissism an issue to be taken seriously by the general public – and not just by psychoanalysts and mental-health professionals.

Vaknin has also come up with some additions to theories on narcissism and how it manifests itself. Perhaps most intriguing is the distinction he draws between somatic narcissists and cerebral narcissists. This helps link our popular notions of narcissists as mirror-hugging dandies with the more worrying implications of how badly narcissists tend to treat other people.

Vaknin says there are two types of narcissist. First, there are those obsessed with their looks, bodies and pulling power. They flaunt everything they have that contributes to their outward magnificence – their possessions, their muscles, their tan, their tattoos, their sexual prowess and exploits. You've seen a lot of them around. They recount their feats of sexual or athletic achievement, but collapse into a gibbering heap when they get the first sniffle of a cold. We're talking about male characteristics really ... but more so. These are somatic narcissists – narcissists who are obsessed with the body.

In contrast, there are the cerebral narcissists – people who build up their sense of magnificence out of an innate feeling of intellectual superiority to everyone else. Cerebral narcissists are arrogant know-alls, who use their knowledge and wit (whether real or imagined) to secure adoration and admiration, in just the same way as somatic narcissists use their looks and physical achievements.

Now this is interesting stuff, because it tunes in with people we all know. Vaknin says it is common for real narcissists to conform to one type – in other words, narcissists tend to be either somatic or cerebral, but somatic narcissists will have times when their behaviour conforms more to the cerebral type, and vice versa. He bases this largely on his own experience. Here's what he says about his own behaviour patterns:

❤

I am a cerebral narcissist. I brandish my brainpower, exhibit my intellectual achievements, bask in the attention given to my mind and its products. I hate my body and neglect it. It is a nuisance, a burden, a derided appendix, an inconvenience, a punishment. Needless to add that I rarely have sex (often years apart) … Invariably, following every life crisis, the somatic narcissist in me took over. I became a lascivious lecher. When this happened, I had a few relationships – replete with abundant and addictive sex – going simultaneously … This outburst of unrestrained, primordial lust waned in a few months and I settled back into my cerebral ways. No sex, no women, no body.

❤

Whether you go with everything Vaknin says or not, there's no doubt he's one of the most outspoken, industrious, fascinating narcissists around.

THE TRUTH ABOUT NARCISSISM

What it all comes down to is this: Narcissism is about everything you thought it was, but more. It's about a natural and in-born self-centredness – the same conviction of one's own centrality to the universe that we see in a thread running from the myth of Narcissus through to the celebrities posing in their beautiful homes in *Hello!* magazine. In infancy, it is a natural means of self-protection.

This should wane as we become adults, in all but extremely stressful situations. But in some people whose sense of self is not well-developed, this doesn't happen. To hide their lack of confidence at dealing with things, they cover up their inner vulnerability by projecting a kind of artificial self. It's a peculiar and malformed type of egotism, which has much in common with the egotism of a child. And it can range from a tendency to self-obsession to highly problematic behaviour patterns that can constitute a personality disorder.

Narcissism is a spectrum of selfishness. It describes something eternal about human beings, because it's about our relationships, both with people and the world around us. It's so fundamental that you can put it into virtually any context. In

Was Sherlock Holmes a narcissist?

Sherlock Holmes has been accused of many things since the death of his creator Sir Arthur Conan Doyle. One recent play revealed that he and his nemesis Moriarty were actually the same person.[11] A novel has fingered him as Jack the Ripper.[12] And many tourists to Baker Street in London have even insisted he's factual.

But now we can reveal that, like many other isolated and cold heroes of detective fiction, he was also a narcissist.

Let's look at the facts. Holmes has few real friends and leads a solitary, inward-looking life – with the distinctly unsociable habits of pipe-smoking and cocaine. His one constant companion, Dr Watson, suits him because he slavishly caters to his whims. Perhaps more significantly, Watson provides him with the means to perpetuate the majesty of his myth – by writing up his exploits for consumption by the wider world.

According to the American commentator on narcissism, Sam Vaknin, the Watsons of this world 'provide the narcissist with an obsequious, unthreatening audience and with the kind of unconditional and unthinking obedience that confirms to him his omnipotence ... They are the perfect backdrop, never likely to attain centre stage and overshadow their master.'[13]

Moreover, Holmes often publicly humiliates Watson, chastising him for being dimwitted. Love and empathy are rarely on display in Holmes – apart from in one particular case, the famous *A Scandal in Bohemia*, where Watson gives an account of the only glimmering of romantic admiration Holmes ever displayed. In fact, it merely serves to illustrate his emotional iciness.

To Sherlock Holmes she is always THE woman. I have seldom heard him mention her under any other name. In his eyes she eclipses and predominates the whole of her sex. It was not that he felt any emotion akin to love for Irene Adler. All emotions, and that one particularly, were abhorrent to his cold, precise but admirably balanced mind. He was, I take it, the most perfect reasoning and observing machine that the world has seen, but as a lover he would have placed himself in a false position. He never spoke of the softer passions, save with a gibe and a sneer. They were admirable things for the observer – excellent for drawing the veil from men's motives and actions.

Holmes is not interested in having relationships with people – he'd rather use them as a source of stimulation for his constantly restless brain. To the narcissistic personality, others can be merely a means to distract, entertain or glorify. And Watson is the main instrument of his manipulation. In *The Adventure of the Copper Beeches*, Holmes coolly criticises Watson for the way he is writing up his accounts of the sleuth's deductive brilliance, putting too much emotion into his records rather than the bare facts.

'It seems to me that I have done you full justice in the matter,' I remarked with some coldness, for I was repelled by the egotism which I had more than once observed to be a strong factor in my friend's singular character.

'No, it is not selfishness or conceit,' said he, answering, as was his wont, my thoughts rather than my words. 'If I claim full justice for my art, it is because it is an impersonal thing – a thing beyond myself...'

Sherlock Holmes had been silent all the morning, dipping continuously into the advertisement columns of a succession of papers until at last, having apparently given up his search, he had emerged in no very sweet temper to lecture me upon my literary shortcomings.

In Sam Vaknin's terms, a classic cerebral narcissist. If he had been around today, Watson would be declaring to the world that he was a victim of narcissistic emotional abuse.

the ethical context, it's about the contrast between selfishness and altruism. In the religious context, it's the contrast between pride and humility. In the social context, it's about individualism and society. In the context of personal relationships, it's about being insensitive or sensitive to another person's needs.

It's on this last, perhaps most practical, aspect that this book focuses, but it will touch on all the other areas in the process. Narcissism is anathema to relationships, which by their very nature cannot revolve around one 'self'. Even in its milder everyday forms, narcissism can cause annoyance that may escalate into larger problems with relationships at home and work. At the more extreme end, it may be ruining your life.

So what effect is narcissism having on you? Read on, and the next chapter will try and help you find out.

Notes

[1] 'So this is George's idea of connecting people and politics?', *The Times,* 14 January 2006.

[2] 'Gav's line-out', the *Sun,* 12 July 2006.

[3] 'Metrosexual, RIP?' Andrew Billen, *The Times*, 7 April 2006.

[4] From *Tales From Ovid*, Met 3, trans. Ted Hughes, Penguin.

[5] Sigmund Freud, *On Narcissism: an introduction,* included in vol. XIV of James Strachey (ed), *The Standard Edition of the Complete Psychological Works of Sigmund Freud*, The Hogarth Press, London,1957.

[6] Marion F Solomon, *Narcissism and Intimacy: love and marriage in an age of confusion*, Norton, New York and London, 1989.

[7] Heinz Kohut, *The Analysis of the Self*, International Universities Press, 1971.

[8] 'Diagnostic Criteria for 301.81 Narcissistic Personality Disorder', *Diagnostic and Statistical Manual of Mental Disorders*, Fourth Edition, American Psychiatric Association, 1994.

[9] Steven Carter and Julia Sokol, *Help! I'm in Love with a Narcissist?*, M Evans and Company Inc., New York, 2005.

[10] www.angelfire.com/zine2/narcissism/malignant_narcissism_vaknin_revisited.html

[11] Jeremy Paul, *The Secret of Sherlock Holmes*, performed at Wyndham's Theatre, 1988–9.

[12] Michael Dibdin, *The Last Sherlock Holmes Story*, Faber and Faber, 1978.

[13] http://samvak.tripod.com/narcissistfriends.html

2
IN THE LOOKING GLASS

Is there a narcissist in your life?

Sonia: 'I love you, Alan.'
Alan Partridge: 'Thanks a lot!'
I'M ALAN PARTRIDGE
BY STEVE COOGAN, ARMANDO IANNUCCI
AND PETER BAYNHAM, 2002

Let's cut to the chase. Is your life being ruined by a narcissist? Let's look at how narcissism manifests itself in our love lives and elsewhere. Could your partner, friends, relations or work colleagues be narcissistic?

Or, more unnervingly, could you be narcissistic? I pose that as a passing point, because if you really were a narcissist you probably wouldn't be reading this. You would have either binned this book already, or concluded that it didn't apply to you – but maybe to your friends and lovers instead. Self-delusion is one of the strongest traits of the true narcissist – the image they have created around themselves renders them largely impervious to self-analysis or criticism. So the main object of this chapter is not to crack the protective shell of genuinely narcissistic personalities. It's really meant as a way of spotting the narcissists around us. But, at the same time, some of us with milder narcissistic traits may recognise something of ourselves in the characteristics described here. If you do, don't call the men in white coats – at least, not for the time being.

Because that's something we've got to bear in mind from the start. Not all narcissists are monsters. In some people this tendency to self-obsession is relatively mild, still allowing other people in. In others, it's severe because the demands of the self are so great that they become hugely problematic.

Propping up one's all-important self-esteem involves creating fantasies about one's own worth, achievements and looks. It requires using other people to reflect glory and worth. The true narcissist needs other people only in so far as they can support their own fantasy image of themselves.

Some psychoanalysts and writers[1] make a distinction between 'healthy narcissism' and 'unhealthy narcissism', with the unhealthy narcissist someone who, no matter what their age, has not yet developed socially or morally, and the healthy narcissist being someone who has a real sense of self-esteem that can enable them to leave their imprint on the world, but who can also share in the emotional life of others.

That may be a bit of an abrupt distinction, but it's worth bearing in mind. For the rest of this book, I'll try to give an indication of which end of the continuum we're talking about, by referring to 'people with narcissistic traits' at the milder end, 'narcissists' towards the middle of the spectrum, and 'narcissistic personalities' at the more extreme end. It's an inexact science – in fact, it's not science at all – but it at least conveys the fact that in some people narcissistic traits are all-consuming, and in others they're not.

Once we begin to recognise narcissistic traits, in ourselves and others, the possibility opens up of beginning to understand previously confusing, and even demeaning, situations. And understanding is the first step to resolving.

Let's start by introducing you to a narcissist called John, recalled by former girlfriend Rosie in her own words. What Rosie has to say demonstrates exactly how narcissists wheedle their way into our hearts, but also how they drive us to distraction.

❤

I'd grown up reading Wuthering Heights *and my romantic ideal was Heathcliff – someone who was volatile and made big gestures. In my teens, my boyfriends were very dull – I thought at the time they'd all become accountants, and actually I was right. I started going out with John when I was nineteen and just starting at art college. I was very idealistic and wanted something real, wanted to be with people who really lived and did real things – though ironically, in the end, that all turned out to be rather false.*

John was exciting because his social background was far less privileged than my own, which meant there was something

rebellious about going out with him. But he also made me feel the ⨍
most special person in the world. That's how narcissists get hold of
you and keep you. I was made to feel special with incredible letters
and poems, and little thoughtful things like him remembering
everything I said I liked, and then weeks, possibly months later,
buying them as presents. I mentioned that I used to collect hippos
as a child, and he went out and bought as many toy and model
hippos as he could find. And I heard from mutual friends that
he talked about me admiringly all the time, which was very
flattering.

John was very good-looking, and lots of people flocked around
him adoringly, and others wanted to be his girlfriend, and that
made me feel very special.

He kept on saying that I would never have another relationship
like this – and I felt that too. The trouble was, I came to realise that
this was his way of keeping me emotionally tied in with him at the
times when his erratic and sometimes cruel behaviour was making
things impossible for me. He was breeding a kind of dependence
that was impossible to live with, because you were constantly up
and down according to his whims. He would take up a persona
and totally live it, and then move on to something else – one week
he'd be into chill music, and the next he'd be totally immersed in
hip hop. Everything was always extreme, and at the beginning that
was very attractive.

But it was complete attention-seeking. We lived in the same
student house, and one day a girlfriend from home came to see me,
but John refused to meet her. He locked himself in the bedroom and

refused to come out. He'd just sneak out when he needed to use the bathroom or get something to eat, but he wouldn't see me until she'd gone, and wouldn't say why he was doing it. He had to be the centre of attention.

And sometimes he had to humiliate me too. He'd have these depressions, where he wouldn't eat anything or talk. He said that if I left his side, he didn't know what he'd do – so of course, I'd stay with him for days on end, during which time he'd be just vile to me. Once John got really angry – I can't remember what it was about, but I think he felt that I was neglecting him, or hadn't understood him. He punched a wall. What was interesting was that he was right-handed, and he punched the wall with his left – it was obviously considered, rather than impulsive, and he was care-ful not to hit himself somewhere that mattered. And he made a point of doing it in my student house, while all my friends were around.

I've read about narcissism since, and I think narcissists behave like this because they want to show that the world revolves around them. If they are nice to you, it's because they want you to love them. That adds to their sense of self-importance. But then they also have to prove that they are better than you, and that you have to be at their beck and call.

So yes, John made me feel wonderful, but he also made me feel absolutely terrible. We were both really into painting, but whenever I painted anything, he said it was rubbish. He was incredibly competitive. I really liked films and knew quite a lot about them, and as soon as we started going out, he had to get into films and become the world's greatest expert on them. He certainly had to prove he knew more than me, and would buy books and swot up.

I don't know what made him the way he was. Maybe it was his family. He hardly ever spoke to his dad, and had no relationship with him. His mother was incredibly close to him, and thought the sun shone out of his arse.

John and I split up after two years, and I didn't see him for three years. Then I called him because I wondered how he was. We met a few times and he wanted to get back together again. He said he'd changed, and part of me wondered whether he had. But then I met him with some of my friends around, and he made it clear he wanted me to himself, and that he didn't want to share me. Then it all came back, and I remembered how he'd been about my friends in the past, and how isolated I felt, and it made me realise that he hadn't really changed at all. I went round to his house and, despite him insisting that we'd get back together one day, I told him that we really were finished. He took me to the station, and my last image was of him weeping hysterically on the platform as my train drew out.

❤

This is a portrait of a narcissist. You can see what a classic case Rosie encountered when you turn to the criteria that American psychiatrists use to identify people they believe have narcissistic personality disorder. They are found in the *American Psychiatric Association's Diagnostic and Statistical Manual of*

Mental Disorders, Fourth Edition – a manual that covers all mental-health disorders for both children and adults.

The manual says that people who have five or more of the following traits can be classed as having a narcissistic personality disorder:

- ♡ has a grandiose sense of self-importance
- ♡ preoccupied with fantasies of unlimited success, power, brilliance, beauty or idealised love
- ♡ believes that they are special and should only associate with special, high-level people
- ♡ needs excessive admiration
- ♡ has a sense of entitlement
- ♡ exploits others
- ♡ lacks empathy
- ♡ envious of others, or thinks they are envious of him
- ♡ haughty, arrogant behaviour.

It's not a pleasant combination, but for all his charms and attractions it fits John like glove. Perhaps his strongest narcissistic traits are as follows:

A preoccupation with fantasises of unlimited brilliance and idealised love

John genuinely believed that Rosie and he constituted something unique and special – no one had ever loved like that, no one could feel stronger, nothing could be more romantic. For

Rosie, however, it eventually became clear that this glamorous image of the romance was illusory because it involved a man who had no genuine interest in how she was feeling, and who depended on humiliating her to make himself feel better.

A belief that he was special and could only be understood by special people

John was very dependent on Rosie, partly because he had singled her out as one of the few people worthy of his attention. Only she could come close to understanding him – that was the key to their great romance. But that didn't mean she was an equal, because, ironically for someone he'd picked out as being special, he was also deeply competitive with her. He had to prove constantly that he was better than her. He needed that to create a sense of self-esteem – something that, deep down, he really didn't have.

Exploiting others

This was not a relationship of equals. Good relationships revolve around being able to maintain one's own sense of self while allowing a partner to manifest their own identity too – preferably with the two of you also boosting each other's sense of self-worth. But John depended on Rosie for his self-esteem, and nothing went the other way. He humiliated her and exploited her in quite a demoralising way. It was the way he propped up his own entirely artificial sense of confidence.

Lacking empathy

It was impossible for John to see things from Rosie's perspective. He couldn't see how infuriating his behaviour was, or how it made Rosie suffer. And it's all because he had created a delusional world where he was centre stage – there's no room for anyone else. Only his own emotions mattered – and his dramatic, but staged, demonstration of anger by hitting a wall is a revealing gesture from a man who could not bear to be ignored by those who should be reflecting his importance.

Envious of others

John wasn't just envious of Rosie, her painting skill, and her interests. He was envious of her friends – and the fact that they might have some sort of hold on Rosie. Because narcissists are so choosy about who to spend time with, they are deeply suspicious and jealous of others who spend time with their chosen ones. Other people are not to be enjoyed or interacted with in their own right – they are either reflectors of grandiosity, or competitors.

That's five out of the list. No doubt, you'll probably now be applying those criteria to yourself and those you know. Fair enough – some of these are traits found to a certain extent in everyone. But do remember (and this is something we'll deal with more in later chapters) that the American Psychiatric Association's checklist of traits was designed to help psychiatrists identify people with a personality disorder characterised by narcissism. And though the list forms a useful baseline for establishing narcissistic behaviour, being able to tick those boxes doesn't necessarily mean that the person has a personality disorder – just one per cent of the population are believed to have an actual narcissistic personality disorder. So let's try to refine the process of characterising narcissists a bit further.

ARE YOU IN A NARCISSISTIC RELATIONSHIP? THE CHECKLISTS

You can use these checklists on behalf of your partner or yourself (if you're self-aware enough). Tick those statements below that tally with your behaviour or that of your partner. I've organised the questions into two groups of ten. The first group of ten questions deals with milder narcissistic traits – the sorts that are found in many people. If you or your partner score five or over in this section, it doesn't necessarily mean you have a major problem, but it does mean that narcissistic traits may be causing unhappiness in your relationship.

People who score over five in the first questionnaire should move on to the second checklist. This itemises more serious narcissistic traits. If you score five or more on this one, it's quite likely that narcissism is ruining your life.

Try to answer the following questions honestly, thinking about examples from your own life that might fit in with the description. But check each time that it really does fit, and it's not just a case of you wanting it to because you've made up your mind already. In phrasing these questions I've assumed, for the sake of convenience, we're talking about a male partner.

Mild narcissistic traits

☐ Does he ever seem to exaggerate his achievements?
For example, will the meal he cooked for you last night be the most fabulous thing you ever tasted when you talk about it the next day (though in fact it was a bit average)?

☐ Does he have a naturally arrogant manner?
Does his haughtiness sometimes make you feel like an inferior being?

☐ Does he expect you to meet his needs, even though he hasn't stated them?
Are you left feeling angry that he has unreasonable expectations of you, for example?

☐ Is he unusually concerned about how others view him?
For example, is he always conscious of 'images' and how he projects himself to the outside world?

☐ When you're together, do you spend more time talking about him than you?

For example, does the conversation always seem to turn away from generalities to specifics about his life?

☐ Is he subject to whims?

For example, will he change his look, his interests and his hobbies at the drop of a hat?

☐ Is he extremely sensitive to criticism?

For example, do you often find yourself forcibly stopping yourself from saying what you think, for fear of how he might react?

☐ Is he obviously flirtatious with other women?

Does he often seem interested in other women, but always insists that you are the only one he could ever love?

☐ Do you feel you have to do most of the work when it comes to keeping the relationship going?

Does it seem that he takes you for granted in a way he never did at the start of your relationship?

☐ Do you feel emotionally drained by how much effort it seems to take to keep your partner happy?

Does he expect that you should do everything?

Serious narcissistic traits

☐ Is there something rather overwhelming about his big romantic gestures?
For example, have you felt a bit suffocated, or been left with an awkward feeling of indebtedness, by the number or expense of presents lavished on you?

☐ Does he show no interest in what you really want, or really feel?
For example, are you often accused of being selfish, when all you are actually doing is trying to convey something about where you fit in to the relationship?

☐ Does he seem to think he's intrinsically better than everyone else?
For example, is he snooty about people who have achieved less than him, or does he get irate when other people are being served in a restaurant before him?

☐ Does he sometimes make you feel like a keeper, rather than a partner?
For example, do you find yourself running round after his smallest wish, or desperately trying to cover up for his antisocial behaviour?

☐ Does his idea of truth and fiction seem very different from yours?

For example, has he ever constructed an entirely fictitious event but insisted it is true?

☐ Do you fear him or fear for him – and stay with him partly because you worry what would happen if you left?

For example, has he ever implied he might fall apart, or even harm himself, if you weren't around?

☐ Have you ever felt your personal safety has been threatened by his thrill-seeking or addictive behaviour?

For example, has he driven erratically and dangerously – seemingly on purpose?

☐ Does he swing from idealising you to treating you as if you're nothing, regardless of what you have done?

For example, are you often left wondering what you have done to suddenly make him hate you so much?

☐ Does he sometimes try to create a rational argument to justify his behaviour, when by any normal standards it is completely unjustifiable?

For example, do you sometimes find yourself wondering whether you're going mad because his idea of normality seems so different from your own?

☐ Do your friends try to tell you he's no good for you?
If you look deep in your heart, are you hiding from what others are telling you about your relationship?

So how did you get on? Does your partner have narcissistic traits? The answers to these questions don't constitute proof, of course. We're all aware of the perils of simple checklists. But they may point you towards some of the reasons why your relationship is not the bed of roses you first expected it to be. If narcissism is affecting your life, in Chapter 5 you'll find an explanation of some of the reasons why people show narcissistic traits, which may help you to understand why your partner behaves as he does. And in Chapters 10 and 11 you'll find advice on some of the practical strategies you might consider to try to address problems of narcissism, and stop it ruining your life.

The examples in the checklist illustrate just how difficult it is to conduct a genuinely meaningful relationship when one of the partners is strongly narcissistic. Narcissism denies the principles of compromise and understanding that are at the base of so many strong partnerships. He needs you. He really does, because you are the means to him having any sense of self-worth. But it's a parasitic kind of need.

NICE NARCISSISTS

Let's take a step back, and look at the results of those two checklists again. Many of you will have scored, say, seven on the first checklist, and two on the second. It doesn't mean you're engaged in a disastrous relationship. It may mean that your partner is extremely nice, with many redeeming features, but that he or she has some narcissistic traits that make life very difficult for you.

In fact, nice narcissists are a common breed – people who, for example, believe that they are driven by compassion, and may have been bolstered in that impression by others, but who within a relationship still expect the world to revolve around them. These types of narcissists can be tricky.

So, in contrast to our earlier examples, which have tended to concentrate on the more extreme end of narcissism, let's look at how it manifested itself in a relationship that showed no outward signs of being unusual or destructive.

❤

Andrew and Hazel have been married for eight years. Before that, they had been going out together for three. Prior to their marriage, and before the couple lived together, everything was a mad romantic whirl – impulse trips abroad (usually at Andrew's instigation), sex on the beach (usually at Hazel's), and nights of laughing, going to glamorous places, and gazing adoringly into each other's eyes. When they married, things started to change. Andrew, a stockbroker, worked long hours, and Hazel noticed that when he wasn't out 'having a good time' he became preoccupied with his work. She also had a high-pressure job at an advertising agency to hold down. But for all the pressures of her work, Andrew expected

Hazel to take the brunt of the household chores, and started to get irate when Hazel reminded him that she was getting increasingly desperate and isolated.

'It wasn't until we started to live together that I realised there was just this expectation that his wants and needs should always come first,' says Hazel. 'I don't think it was even a conscious thing on Andrew's part. He was always very popular with people, and had this aura of personableness and of being kind. That was one of the things that drew me to him. But there was something deep inside him that just couldn't get outside of his head and into mine, to see how hard he was making it for me when, say, he just expected to be able to be out as late as he liked with his friends after work.

'Things got so much worse when we had our first son, Joe, because the pressures on me obviously got considerably worse, especially after I returned to work and Joe went to nursery. We had constant arguments. I think Andrew genuinely wanted to try to be sympathetic – because that's the image he had of himself. But when it came down to it, he had no inner mechanisms for thinking of how I felt or reminding himself that every time he put his own wishes first – from what to watch on television, to where we went on holiday, and who picked up Joe in the evenings. It was as if he lived in a fantasy world where everything was fine, and he could do whatever he wanted, and all those messy, difficult bits of life would just get done.

'It wasn't just a matter of me being unsupported. He was constantly demanding more from me, even though I couldn't cope as it was. If I was trying to fix Joe's food, he'd start having a *go that we weren't feeding the child properly, or that I left the kitchen in a tip and it was unhygienic. And then he'd go on about feeling unsupported himself, about how I never made love to him any more, or asked him about his work, or made a fuss of him on his birthday like I used to. Sometimes he used to deliberately bug me to gain attention – for example, bombarding me with emails when he knew I was up against a deadline on a really important piece of work.'*

The rows got worse and worse, and then were followed by weeks of silences as Hazel realised that no matter what she said, Andrew was incapable of empathising with her, or remembering that he had to fundamentally change his behaviour to make her life more bearable. Eventually, she got Andrew to agree to them both going to a marriage counsellor.

'It was hard for both of us, but I think it was especially hard for Andrew because he was having to wake up to something that was very fundamental to his make-up – his lack of empathy – which conflicted significantly with the image of himself he'd built up since his childhood of being kind and considerate. Things are much better between us now – but it's not that Andrew's changed. He's just more aware of what he tends to do, so when I pull him up over stuff, he can't just dismiss it any more. And he makes a real effort not to make himself the centre of attention any more. He knows there's a certain jealousy thing going on with Joe, that's he's competing with him for my attention, and he hates that and is really working on it.'

♥

This is how a lot of men behave. It's not pathological, and it's not terribly dramatic. But it is something that can be described as narcissistic.

NARCISSISM AND SELFISHNESS

So are we just talking about old-fashioned selfishness? The case of Andrew certainly sounds like selfishness. And if narcissism is such an important character trait, then why has the word only come into widespread use recently? Didn't people used to be referred to as just 'selfish' instead, and cause exactly the same problems in relationships as narcissists? We all know about selfish lovers, unable to think of the gratification of their partner but only of their own.

It's a legitimate point, because it raises the whole question of whether our attitude to words like 'narcissism' partly depends on whether we live in times when imposing the self is something that's applauded or frowned upon by society – something that we'll be looking at in much more detail in Chapter 6. In today's individualistic age, the word 'selfishness' is disappearing, because looking after the self, rather than looking after society, is often expected of us. Perhaps 'narcissism' is taking its place, because we're more interested in personal psychology and diagnostic labels than society.

But narcissism is more than selfishness. It's a particular form of selfishness that requires the attention of others to feed it – almost like human oxygen. Selfishness implies a wilful imposition of self, but narcissism is more of an involuntary imposition – because it's a manifestation of personality, not will. Narcissists really can't help being self-centred. They are simply unable to empathise with others.

PERSONALITY TYPES

Let's look at how you identify a narcissist from a slightly different angle: in terms of personalities. If you use the criteria from the American Psychiatric Association mentioned earlier, it's easy to look at narcissism as some sort of illness, when in fact it's a description of complex human characteristics. It's just as useful to look at narcissism in terms of how our characters are formed. Because if we're acknowledging that narcissism is an intrinsic part of the human make-up – a kind of primitive survival mechanism that gets adjusted and repressed as we sub-consciously learn the necessity of fitting in with others and making partnerships – it's fair enough to assume that some of us are bound to be more narcissistic than others.

This is what Freud believed, and the personality grouping that follows, based on his work, presents narcissism less as something problematic than as an intrinsic part of all human nature. Freud was one of the first thinkers on the human psyche to categorise our personalities into types. His early work on character types[2] gave rise to the 'anal character'. It's a phrase that has stuck in popular parlance – people who are uptight and sticklers for detail are still referred to as 'anal types'. But Freud's character types go deeper than that, and reflect on how narcissism develops, and how it moulds our characters – ideas that were taken further by the psychoanalysts and psychologists that followed him.

It is in our childhood that our basic characters are moulded, and where the roots lie for many of the problems that people like Andrew and John exhibit. The earliest factors that determine a child's eventual personality are obviously the genes that they are born with. But they are also determined by the way they are cared for and educated. Young children who are nurtured in different ways will end up with different characters. Children who live in a threatening environment and who have unsympathetic or emotionally absent parents are less likely to develop the kinds of resilient personalities that will help them cope with the challenges society throws at them as they grow up.

Freud categorised different stages of the child's development, and different types of personality, according to what happened to children during these vital developmental states. He called these libidinal types. According to Freud, the libido is a type of instinctive energy that all human beings have when they are born – a type of life force, if you like. This goes through various phases as we mature, determining people's personalities as it develops. According to what happened during childhood, people are either more or less likely to develop the attributes of certain libidinal types – either getting stuck at one point in the libido's development, or moving on to the next.[3]

Freud came up with three libidinal types, or personality

groups. Each group, as a result of their upbringing, has a very different reaction to the 'socialising' forces we encounter as we grow up. None of us should look to conform too neatly to these types, but they do usefully reflect the fact that we all respond to situations of stress, love and society quite differently. There have been other groupings of personality type put together by psychologists, but Freud's categories neatly capture some of the most distinctive traits of narcissists.

So here are the three types, with some of the characteristics Freud attributed to them. Below each are ten key questions, which may help you pinpoint which one applies to you or your partner. Tick each point that applies to you, or to the person you are answering on behalf of.

The erotic

This group is highly focused on love: loving, but more importantly being loved, is the most important thing in their life. They are governed by the dread of loss of love, which makes them very dependent on those who may withhold love from them.

- ☐ Do you value friends and family, and depend on them to provide security?
- ☐ Do you tend to bring people together?
- ☐ Do you find being on your own hard?
- ☐ Do you think you sometimes show your emotions too much?

☐ Do you sometimes think you are too trusting?
☐ Do you fear conflict?
☐ Do you try to encourage others to collaborate?
☐ Do you hate the idea of people not liking you?
☐ Do you find it hard to make tough decisions?

The obsessional

Rather than being dependent on the people around them, as erotics are, people in this group are very self-reliant, and are guided by worries about what might be the right thing to do. They are naturally conservative, sticklers for detail, and upholders of existing institutions rather than innovators.

☐ Do you set yourself high ideals that you try to live up to?
☐ Are you diligent?
☐ Are you a stickler for timekeeping?
☐ Are you obsessive about tidiness?
☐ Are you choosy about your friends, but tend to be loyal?
☐ Do you set about completing tasks in a very systematic way?
☐ Are you resistant to change?
☐ Do you get upset if things are not done the right way?
☐ Are you judgemental?

The narcissistic

Love is not a prime influence for members of this group – their main interest is self-preservation. Narcissists are independent and not easily overawed. They can strike others as being 'personalities' and often want to change things radically.

☐ Do you only trust your own opinions?
☐ Do you sometimes think the world is conspiring against you?
☐ Do you think people are either for you or against you?
☐ Are you competitive?
☐ Do you voraciously want to learn things?
☐ Are you very sensitive to criticism?
☐ Do you tend not to listen to others?
☐ Do you tend to exaggerate?
☐ Do others find you a bit grandiose?
☐ Do you have a strong vision of how things should be, and want to change everything to fit?

INTERPRETING THE RESULTS

You may well find that you (or the person you are answering on behalf of) don't clearly fall into one category – you're most likely to have a personality that bestrides two of these groups. This is typical. Mixed types are far more common than pure types – reflecting the fact that human beings aren't easily classifiable caricatures. Freud commented that erotic-obsessionals, erotic-narcissists, and narcissistic-obsessionals really do reflect the personalities of many people encountered by psychotherapists. Here are the characteristics of the crossover groups:

Erotic obsessionals

Dependent on those currently close to them, but also dependent on those who have created a sense of order for them in the past, such as parents and educators. This gives them their sense of security. They are generally systematic people who want to help others, but worry about being loved.

Erotic narcissists

Perhaps the most common group, where the contrasting attitudes of narcissists and obsessionals towards love and dependence cancel each other out. They are generally creative people who are poor on the details.

Narcissistic obsessionals

Culturally very valuable people, because they have a resilient independence, but act out of conscience, and do so with great vigour. They are generally people who at their best can be charismatic yet practical, and at their worst are controlling and paranoid.

You'll see a lot in this personality-typing that tallies with the characteristics of narcissists pinpointed in our earlier checklists. What's different here is that narcissistic characteristics are very much integrated into the human personality as a whole. Freud and his followers in the field of psychoanalysis and psychology have not necessarily viewed narcissism as bad. It simply exists. Indeed, the leading American psychoanalyst and business consultant, Michael Maccoby (to whom I should acknowledge a debt for inspiring the above questionnaire), believes that the natural energy and individuality of narcissists is the key to much industrial progress and innovation. As we'll see in Chapters 6 and 7, narcissism is a strong and sometimes positive influence on society.

Narcissistic characteristics can also make some men very easy to fall in love with, as we'll see in the next chapter. Unfortunately, on the whole such men are not very good at long-term relationships. Indeed, the more plentiful the strands of narcissism in a personality, the more difficult that personality is likely to be for those in close proximity. Of all the personality types, the most narcissistic are the most emotionally isolated. As Hazel and Rosie found, that can make them a nightmare to love.

Notes

[1] Sandy Hotchkiss, *Why is it Always About You? The seven deadly sins of narcissism*, Free Press, New York, 2002.

[2] Sigmund Freud, *Character and Anal Eroticism*, 1908, included in

James Strachey (ed), *The Standard Edition of the Complete Psychological Works of Sigmund Freud*, The Hogarth Press, London, 1957.

3 Sigmund Freud, *Libidinal Types*, 1931, included in James Strachey (ed), *The Standard Edition of the Complete Psychological Works of Sigmund Freud*, The Hogarth Press, London, 1957.

3

ENTER MR DARCY

Why it's easy to fall in love with narcissists

Every night when I go off to bed and when I wake up
I want you I want you
I'm going to say it again 'til I instil it
I know I'm going to feel this way until you kill it
I want you I want you
ELVIS COSTELLO, 'I WANT YOU'

And now for some romantic fiction. It's given a certain twist by romantic fact.

❤

His friend Mr Darcy soon drew the attention of the room by his fine, tall person, handsome features, noble mien, and the report which was in general circulation within five minutes after his entrance, of his having ten thousand a year. The gentlemen pronounced him to be a fine figure of a man, the ladies declared he was much handsomer than Mr Bingley, and he was looked at with great admiration for about half the evening, till his manners gave

a disgust which turned the tide of his popularity; for he was dis-
covered to be proud; to be above his company, and above being
pleased.[1]

❤

Let's start by making it clear that Mr Darcy was not a narcissist. He wasn't because, as we all know (or at least need to believe), he and Elizabeth Bennet fell permanently in love, and, despite his rather grumpy demeanour, lived happily ever after. On the whole, things aren't that simple with narcissists.

But what is interesting about Mr Darcy is that the very qualities that have made him the object of feminine drooling since the eighteenth century are the very qualities that can make narcissists so appealing to women. Narcissistic men often display the classic archetypal characteristics of the male romantic hero.

Let's have a look at that description of Mr Darcy. Handsome and clearly conscious of his appearance. Proud, giving the appearance of being above everyone else. Emotionally self-contained, and not easily displaying pleasure.

Now let's look at some of the characteristics of the narcissistic personality, as defined by the American Psychiatric Association: 'grandiose sense of self-importance', 'requires excessive admiration', 'shows arrogant, haughty behaviors or attitudes'. Some resemblance there. And what is it about Darcy that really makes Elizabeth Bennet fall in love with him? It's not his haughty attitude in itself, which partly repels her. It is a side to him that no one else can see – beneath the pride, she discerns a sensitivity and vulnerability. And it is, of course, only revealed to her.

❤

'I do, I do like him,' she replied, with tears in her eyes, 'I love him. Indeed he has no improper pride. He is perfectly amiable. You do not know what he really is; then pray do not pain me by speaking of him in such terms.'[2]

❤

There's that sense that only the two lovers can see the real person beneath their external veneers, and it's a classic characteristic of the intoxicating romantic relationship. Look no further than *Jane Eyre* and *Wuthering Heights* for more examples of dark, impenetrable types who will reveal their true soul only to the heroine, and heroines who feel they are the only person who can save this tortured soul.

Those trusted romantic ingredients are fundamental to the way relationships with narcissists start. Narcissistic men exude a sense of vulnerability, mystery and unpredictability. They know it, and often pride themselves on their ability to attract women like moths to an open flame. 'I think one of the ways I got hooked into the relationship is that Roger made me feel as if I was the only person on the planet that understood him,' says Nancy, 33, who has struggled in a relationship with Roger – a man she now recognises as a narcissist – for eight years. 'That's quite a powerful thing, because it puts one in a position of real responsibility. It certainly made me become more accepting of some of his more extreme behaviour because early on he'd drummed into me that he was different and in some way special.'

Talking to women who have fallen in love with a narcissist, it's amazing how many mention the Heathcliff Factor. We have already heard, in Chapter 2, from Rosie, who said that her romantic ideal was the hero of *Wuthering Heights* – she wanted someone real and a bit wild who lived life to the full, unlike the rather dull youths who had courted her in her teenage years.

Now here's more from Nancy, who reveals not just why it's easy to fall in love with men like this, but why the traits that make them into a bit of a romantic hero can also make them difficult to leave. It's like being an adrenaline junkie.

♥

He appeals to a certain kind of woman – and I count myself among them. It's the Heathcliff thing. I think women find that kind of man attractive for a number of reasons. First of all, they think 'If only he was with me he'd change'. It's a sort of Beauty and the Beast story – only you can turn the monster into a handsome prince. Second, when Roger shines his light on someone, it makes them feel very special. I suppose it's partly because he doesn't do it very often.

♥

Anyone recognise a bit of Darcy in that? She went on to tell me:

❤

When you've had a relationship with someone with those traits, it's very difficult to have anything else. It's like living life at a different volume. Other men don't seem as exciting or as tangible as Roger. There's just something. He looked at me in a way no one before or since has ever done. It's part fear, it's part flattery – it almost feels as if nothing could ever feel that safe, or that exciting, again.

❤

These are the characteristics of men that women have found alluring for centuries. They are classic manifestations of the narcissistic personality. Women are drawn into relationships with narcissistic men who, by their very nature, are very difficult to relate to long-term – because their outlook is so centred on the self that they find it extremely difficult to have insight into other people's feelings. It adds up to a one-way-street relationship that isn't going anywhere.

THE MAN WHO SWEEPS A WOMAN OFF HER FEET

Let's look in a bit more detail about what it is in narcissistic men that can make women go weak at the knees. We have the brooding male, and the woman who is the only one who can see the real man. Let's add another classic Mills & Boon ingredient: the whirlwind romance. The man lavishes attention on the woman that no one else could: flowers on the pillow, trips to Paris, abundant compliments. It's so romantic, so intense … perhaps too intense.

Here's an account from Shelley, another woman who fell in love with a narcissist, and who recounted her experiences on an internet site for victims of male narcissists:

♥

He was the most charming, romantic, witty, charismatic and handsome man I had ever met. I had never before been so attracted to someone. I was completely in his thrall. He called me all the time, texted me continuously, declared his love perpetually. We walked in rhythm, we fitted together like jigsaw pieces. The sex was a spiritual experience. I suddenly knew what Hollywood was all about; I felt that my new romance was like something from the silver screen, a veritable fairytale. Then the hell happened. It has taken me ages to recover.

♥

There are hundreds of similar accounts from women who are now seeing themselves as victims not of the classic male bastard, but of a particular type of male bastard. They are men who are romantic heroes for a while, and then prove themselves emotionally incapable – those big romantic gestures that at first proved so alluring are in fact the whole deal, symptomatic of these men's need to show off and be the centre of attention. Once the initial gloss of the relationship wears off, they display an inability to understand the world of others. They are too bound up with their own world.

But it's so hard to resist. When we want to be loved, big acts of seeming devotion can make us feel more special than anything else. Here's some more from Nancy. Some of Roger's romantic acts during their courtship are straight out of a Hollywood movie.

❤

Once, soon after I'd met him, he drove 200 miles to deliver me some fish and chips. I was at my flat at home in London, and he was up in Blackpool at some conference. I was talking to him on the phone – I couldn't go out because I had a bad cold and I said something about really fancying fish and chips, and how lucky he was to be by the seaside. And he drove all the way down to London, with this rather soggy fish and chips wrapped up in goodness knows how many newspapers, rang the doorbell, and left it on the doorstep for me with a note. Then he drove all the way back without even seeing me. He was master of the Grand Gesture.

❤

But the full story of their relationship reveals another side to such big displays. If they were about declaring love, fine. If they were about other things, they could be disturbing.

♥

It didn't take me that long to realise that he was capable of doing extreme things the other way too. Just as the fish and chips was a grand romantic gesture, weeks afterwards he performed the destructive gesture of deliberately cutting his arm with a kitchen knife. He was feeling neglected because I'd been fifteen minutes on the phone to another man, and I think he thought I was flirting outrageously. Maybe I was.

♥

Roger is clearly an extreme case. But there are thousands of others without such deep problems whose allure for women is bound up with the qualities that make them deeply difficult. Here is another account, this time from a woman contributing to a discussion forum for women who feel they are victims of male narcissists:

♥

When we met he was the most wonderful person I had ever known. He was funny, charming, independent, and fulfilled all of my emotional and physical needs, but after a few months things began to change. I could not figure out what was going on. It was like he was a totally different person. I did everything to make things work.

♥

AN ALLURING WORLD

There's another characteristic of narcissists that tends to attract people romantically: their fantasy world. Whereas Mr Darcy actually does have a lot to be proud about – his wealth, his abilities, his well-hidden but genuine compassion – narcissists can create the alluring impression of these to build their sense of self-esteem. In fact, they're fabricated. Some narcissists believe themselves to be on a par with celebrities and other high achievers – so they will always want to be seen in the right circles, with the right people and in the right places. They'll make sure they're seen moving in a glamorous, high-flying world – hanging out at the best bars, clubs, restaurants, and spurning the places frequented by mere commoners.

American relationships authors Steven Carter and Julia Sokol have pointed out that such personality-types can also emulate the charitable nature of many celebrities. Some want to be Albert Schweitzer, or Mother Teresa. 'Narcissists are just as likely to be found working for charity organizations building homes for the impoverished as they are in large corporate offices,' they say.[3]

Now what could be more appealing to the opposite sex than someone who's made a success of himself but cares for the downtrodden? It's irresistible. That seeming self-confidence combined with an ability to share and feel is the stuff of a million matinée idols. And it's exactly what narcissists display. When it all proves to be a veneer, then you know you've fallen in love with a narcissist.

ARE ALL NARCISSISTS MEN?

You'll have noticed that I've been talking about romantic stereotypes of the male all this time. There is a reason for this, which will be developed in the chapters that follow. Although there are many women who are narcissists, the current estimate among psychoanalysts is that up to three-quarters of narcissists are male. Scan the literature, talk to the people who feel they've been victims of narcissists, and you'll find the vast majority of case studies are about men. The qualities of the narcissist tie in very closely with the male, and the traditional concept of the macho romantic lead.

Of course, women have always been mocked by men in the past for their narcissism in the general sense of being vain. And there are now women coming forward and declaring themselves to be narcissists in the more complex, egotistical sense. But they are a minority, and arguably becoming a smaller one as men display increasing signs of the physical vanity that was once meant to be the trademark of women.

So when we talk about narcissism, are we simply talking about natural male traits? After all, those characteristics that have been pinned down by the American Psychiatric Association as narcissistic – grandiosity, lack of empathy, ruthlessness, arrogance – sound surprisingly like a personality profile of the more testosterone-laden specimens of manhood. Well, yes and no. Yes, in that those influences that seem to determine how narcissistic people are – their genes, their upbringing and other environmental triggers – are the same influences that determine whether you're an ultra male or a more feminine type. And yes, in that there seems to be something quite deeply rooted in men's fundamental sexual make-up that makes narcissistic relationships – egotistical, emotionally detached men having relationships with subservient women – somehow a romantic archetype. It's the James Bond male fantasy. One of the theories of why high-achieving women find it so hard to get partners is that some men find that kind of equality hard – they want someone to feed their own sense of importance, not someone who can challenge them and take centre stage.

But no, in that narcissism isn't a prerequisite of being male, and being a woman doesn't make you exempt. Many of the reasons that women fall in love with male narcissists will also be the reasons that men fall in love with female narcissists. But men, in all their vulnerable, infuriating, excluding and occasionally glorious self-centredness, do tend to exemplify narcissism – and I'll be dealing with these gender issues in a bit more detail in Chapter 5.

But what does all this tell us about romance? Why on earth should women be so susceptible to the charms of men who will often make their lives difficult, where their own personalities will be in danger of being subsumed? After all, most women can spot a cheat and a liar from 200 paces – if they don't happen to fall in love with them, that is.

There are some very good reasons why women fall for narcissistic types, and I'm going to concentrate on three of them.

First, it's partly the nature of romance that we are drawn to people whose vulnerabilities dovetail with our own. We are attracted to people who need us as well as want us. And narcissists are some of the neediest people around.

Second, women may be hard-wired to fall in love with strong, domineering and erratic types because, according to some theorists, it holds an evolutionary advantage.

Third, many women are vulnerable to narcissistic men because they themselves come from a background where narcissism was normal – and so those sorts of traits subconsciously feel 'right'.

Let's look at each of the reasons for women's particular susceptibility to this type of man.

Susceptible because of the nature of romance

Falling in love is itself a narcissistic process. There's something in all of us that wants to find a partner who reflects ourselves. Researchers have demonstrated that humans find partners who are actually genetically very similar to themselves. J Philippe Rushton, a psychologist at the University of Western Ontario, found that similar genetics accounted for about one-third of criteria we unconsciously use in selecting a partner.[4] Liliana Alvarez from the Universidad Simón Bolívar in Venezuela authored a significant paper in the *Journal of Evolutionary Psychology* in 2005, indicating that we actually choose mates who look like us.[5] After conducting experiments analysing photographs of couples, she concluded that choosing someone who looks like you is a good means of finding a partner with 'good' genes, but who is not related – optimising the chances of offspring surviving. We really do look for people who mirror ourselves.

But beyond the biology, there are other ways that love is naturally narcissistic. Relationships are all about vulnerability. We often look for people who can try to fill areas where we feel inwardly empty – someone, for example, who can provide the love for ourselves that we ourselves cannot generate, for whatever reason. In doing so, we often find people who themselves have a need to be needed – people who also want an emptiness filled.

This interdependence when falling in love isn't unusual – in fact, some would say it's what romance is all about. There's an emotional 'fit' that people often find with each other, based on their needs, or neediness. This seems to play a big part in the way many romantic relationships start off. Being totally unable to contemplate life without the other person, to be completely dependent on their attention, is, after all, part and parcel of love. The problem is that it's very difficult, in the context of this euphoric sense of oneness and fulfilling each other's needs, to tell how deep the neediness really goes. To tell, indeed, whether the dependency of at least one of the partners has its roots in a severe narcissistic vulnerability.

Let's look at a typical romantic fantasy. Here's Ali talking about the first few weeks of her relationship with Sebastian, when she was eighteen and he was twenty-one:

♥

I had huge rows with my mum and dad. They were worried about me because he was older, and he came from a very different social background. He came from a very well-to-do family. They also thought he was a bit of a waster – he'd never gone to college, or got a job, just played in a band. I thought he was fabulous, and said all the typically teenage things – which part of me still thinks are true. I said they didn't understand how much we loved each other, and that I'd change him. I said that we were really good for each other, because we made each other so happy. And yes, I said it was only with him that I felt alive, because it was true – he really did give me something that no one else ever had.

♥

It's a typical account of an argument that's been conducted in a million living rooms. What Ali recounts is how it feels to fall in love. It's fabulous because the mutual adoration gives one a feeling of being uniquely loved – just as you were as a baby, before any idea of being separate from your mother entered your head. In fact, some psychoanalysts, like Marion F Solomon, believe that in the first bloom of a romantic relationship, the lovers subconsciously believe that their partner can repair or compensate for any lack of love in their early upbringing.[6]

If you talk to relationship counsellors, they'll tell you that this euphoric state invariably doesn't last as a relationship progresses. How could it? You simply can't live life like that. And you can't change people either, at least not by yourself. Normally, as a relationship settles down, it moves on to a stage where the lovers subconsciously realise that they aren't joined at the hip, and don't expect the other to repair emotional damage single-handedly. They are separate human beings, with different needs and desires which potentially conflict. And in healthy relationships, both partners recognise the independence of the other, adjusting their behaviour and constantly trying to take into account the other person's individuality. This isn't always easy, and in many less mature relationships it doesn't happen so well. One or both partners can get worried about the end of a feeling of 'oneness', and feel it is indicative of a deteriorating relationship. They might feel threatened, and put up all sorts of defensive strategies to protect their own individuality.

However, in relationships where there is a narcissistic partner, these latter eventualities become far more likely, and serious. People who are narcissistically vulnerable have an inbuilt sensitivity to being hurt emotionally, and their fear of hurt or humiliation is so great that they find the idea of the 'oneness' of a relationship beginning to change into something different quite frightening. They subconsciously look to their romantic partner to be able to provide everything they lack – someone who can be part of them. To psychoanalysts, they are almost childlike, seeking to be uniquely loved, as a baby is by its mother. The inevitable realisation that lovers are actually separate individuals is very hard indeed for a true narcissist to contemplate.

So it's not entirely surprising that many women end up with a different sort of man than the one they first met. They fall in love, as all of us do, and believe in total dependency and oneness. Narcissists present that sense of romantic oneness beautifully, because it's what they really believe in. The trouble is, they have no concept of the opposite – of independence, other people's individuality and wants and needs. When the partner wants the relationship to move on, as it inevitably must, the narcissist cannot. That spells conflict.

That's exactly what happened with Ali. Despite all her protestations that this was true love that would last, five months after her argument with her mum and dad her relationship with Sebastian was over. If he hadn't had such strong narcissistic tendencies, it might have lasted – they might have been able to work through their differences, and get round the fact that Ali had to go to university and start living her own life. As it was, he couldn't deal with the idea that she wouldn't always be around for him, or that he'd have to share her with other people. 'It was that, more than anything else, he couldn't bear,' says Ali. 'It was that I would start to make new friends. He really started playing up, and was quite horrible to me, saying that I'd hate it at university and never fit in.' It ended when Sebastian told her that he was also going out with one of Ali's old friends – but Ali thinks he did it mainly for effect. The last words she said to him were 'I hate you'. But she still thinks he's the love of her life.

Susceptible by upbringing

Psychologists and psychoanalysts believe there may be another reason why some women are attracted to narcissistic men – and the answer lies in their upbringing. Women who have themselves come from a background where their parents and caregivers have been detached, and expected the world to revolve around them, may be more likely to find narcissistic traits desirable in a man.

Think about it. If your mum or your dad showed some strong narcissistic characteristics – for example, if they expected you to look after them rather than the other way around, or if they expected you to always follow their agenda, or if they found it hard to empathise with your wants and needs – then those sorts of traits would assume a kind of normality. You would have an unspoken expectation that that's just how families are. So when you meet someone who has similar traits to your parents, who, say, expects everyone else to follow their own agenda, it doesn't necessarily seem strange or threatening: at least at first. In fact, it can feel quite familiar, even comforting.

So women who have had an upbringing that was not centred on them can be especially susceptible to getting into relationships with narcissists. This doesn't necessarily mean that their parents were narcissistic monsters. It's all a matter of degree. As I've said earlier, narcissism is evident in all of us to some extent. Behaviour that isn't cruel on the part of parents but verges on the self-centred will not necessarily set up a disastrous cycle in their child. But there is at least some anecdotal evidence that it may make their children more susceptible to the charms of people who are themselves narcissists.

Even if we don't fully understand the reasons why some women seem to be more attracted to narcissistic men than others, it is reasonable to consider the possibility that it is an emotional vulnerability of some sort that aligns their poles to the particular magnetic draw of narcissistic men. This isn't bad – it's just how humans are. We all have our weak points.

Nancy has her own interpretation of why Roger continues to have such power over her:

❤

I don't really know whether I'm particularly susceptible to someone like him. I know that everyone's a product of their experiences. And someone who has a healthy sense of self is less likely to be taken in. When I realised what the problem with Roger was, I read the narcissism message boards on the internet obsessively and lots of the people there were very fragile. But some weren't.

❤

Perhaps Roger spotted her sense of vulnerability, and saw that it would allow him to have some extra hold on her.

❤

There was one really powerful incident. I'd told Roger about some of the more difficult aspects of my childhood, and the next time I saw him, he turned up with a huge box filled with all sorts of childish things, teddy bears, sweets, toys and told me that he was going to make up for everything that had happened in the past. In a way it was a bit like the knight in shining armour thing.

❤

Susceptible by nature

There could be another reason why women are so prone to the double-edged charms of a narcissist. They may have evolved to be that way. There is a theory that women have evolved to respond favourably to signals of grandiosity, self-sufficiency and arrogance given off by men – just the sorts of messages that narcissists specialise in sending out. So they could be programmed to fall in love with narcissistic men.

The theory is called the evolutionary theory of mate selection, and it works like this. Looking at things from a purely scientific and evolutionary point of view, we know that both men and women are looking for the same thing when selecting a partner – someone who is likely to give them healthy offspring who will be able to flourish into adulthood. That way, there are the best chances of lots of surviving offspring, and therefore of the species flourishing.

So from prehistory onwards, men and women have picked up on signals from the opposite sex to indicate that they are a good option on the breeding front. It's the human equivalent of a peahen being attracted to the peacock with the biggest, glossiest and least-damaged feathers, because this indicates they are well-nourished and fit, and strong enough to fight off other males without too much damage. All of which implies that their sperm are probably quite fit too.

Human beings don't have feathers, so we pick up on other signals. The theory is – and most of the work on this has been done by David Buss, a psychology professor at the University of Texas – that in general, males look for signals that suggest fertility, and females look for signals that suggest high status and economic security. This makes sense because in the live-hard-die-young days of prehistory, the best way a male could guarantee the continuation of the species was to mate with as many fertile women as possible (we are talking centuries ago here), while for a woman the best way was to have a safe and secure environment that would allow the few children she was likely to have to be raised safely.

So what a man is looking for is rather simple: youth and beauty, because at a superficial level they are the most accurate indicators of health and fertility (fertility in women declines rapidly with age).

For women, it's a bit more tricky. Yes, general appearance of a male will at least give some indication of their status – a scrawny scruff is probably not your best bet financially. But in the absence of glossy feathers, women have to look for other qualities that give an accurate indication of whether they're going to be good providers. Social and evolutionary psychologists like Buss suggest that women are drawn to cues indicating availability of resources, dominance, high social status, ambition and anything that indicates success.[7]

So in addition to sussing out whether the man owns a Maserati, a second home in Cape Cod and a shelf full of athletics trophies, a woman will be subconsciously assessing a man's air of superiority, whether he has an arrogance born of success.

From the perspective of narcissism, this is extremely interesting. It suggests that those qualities that narcissists tend to display are actually those that women are programmed to look out for in a mate. The aura of success might be real or concocted. As we'll see in Chapter 6, if the circumstances are right, narcissistic men can be highly rich and successful, but in others the signals of arrogance, success and superiority are deceptive – not a sign of real status, but an elaborate and self-deceiving bluff to conceal an inner sense of inadequacy. But whether the arrogance is based on nothing or on real achievements, it still hits an emotional chord in many women. It says: *breed with me.*

Remember that this theory revolves around natural selection. It's not a conscious thought process that women go through, thinking, 'Phwoar, I fancy him because he looks as if he's a real high achiever.' It's just an inbuilt part of the way she desires a mate, like other intrinsic aspects of our personality. And the fact is that in the twenty-first century, it may have entirely outgrown its usefulness. Men's and women's brains are the way they are because throughout our evolution, the types of brains best adapted to breeding have been more likely to survive and multiply, leaving the brains that are less likely to produce offspring to die out. It's worked just fine to make human beings the success story they are today. The trouble is that evolution is a very long process, and our moral standards and social structures change faster than our brains. However, narcissism is possibly a vestige of our more primitive selves, which still figures strongly in the male make-up and in female attraction as a result of that. There will be more about this in Chapter 5.

THE WIT TO WOO

What about those other qualities of narcissists that the women I spoke to found so alluring – those big romantic gestures, that exciting sense of unpredictability and originality, that sense of fun? Geoffrey Miller, an evolutionary psychologist from the Department of Psychology at the University of New Mexico, has something very interesting to say on this.[8]

Remember Rosie, who didn't want to go out with the accountant types who were just so, well, boring. She fell for John, a man who kept on changing his appearance, who depended on her, humiliated her, and couldn't bear the attention to be on anyone but himself – but who she found intensely attractive because he was somehow different, unpredictable, creative. Miller says there's an evolutionary reason why these qualities are so alluring. In primitive societies random behaviour and appearance would bring strategic advantages both in out-witting opponents and avoiding being preyed upon by animals. Regularity of habits and predictable behaviour could all too easily lead to capture. That meant that a strain of natural un-predictability in men might be to their advantage – they were likely to be better hunters, better at fighting off opponents and generally more successful.

Women who were attracted to these qualities would have been at an advantage – they were more likely to end up with successful men, who could provide for them and their offspring. In turn, that meant that their female offspring were likely to have similar preferences, and so, by natural selection, many women came to naturally fancy men with an element of un-predictability.

Miller says that this successful strain of impulsivity – what he calls 'social proteanism' – in men gave rise to all sorts of other qualities we now value in society. He says it may have laid the genetic foundations for 'creative courtship', or what he wryly coins 'the wit to woo'. Amusing and unpredictable romantic behaviour, he says, would have become a reliable indicator to women of men's ability to dodge sabre-toothed tigers. So sexual selection favoured minds prone to inventing imaginative fantasies, and fantastically adventurous things to do together.

You may call all of this romance, and that's exactly what it is. It's just that love can lead us down some strange pathways as well as some glorious ones, and the pathway that leads to highly narcissistic men – experts in the field of fantasy and romance – can be intensely problematic. Could Mr Darcy have been one of those narcissistic men who initially floored women, but turned out to be deeply needy of constant attention and lacking in understanding of others? It would only be revealed when the initial romantic rush of his relationship with Elizabeth wore off. And, sadly, Jane Austen never provided us with a sequel.

Was Lord Byron a narcissist?

Lord Byron, the nineteenth-century poet and adventurer, was responsible for the very picture of romantic heroes that prevails to this day. It wasn't just through the characters he created, such as Childe Harold and Don Juan, but through his own image – saturnine, enigmatic and supposedly 'mad, bad and dangerous to know' (his lover Caroline Lamb's famous assessment). He was prepared to die for a cause he believed in, and he had an amazing power over women. After the success in 1812 of his second book of poems, which sold out within days, he became the original pop celebrity, with women falling over themselves to be near him, and his private life was constantly invaded by fans trying to catch a glance of their idol. His life was a riot of indulgence (he claimed to have slept with 250 women in Venice in the course of one year), ending when he died of fever while fighting with the Greeks in their war of independence.

Some commentators have suggested his extreme and often unpredictable behaviour had its origins in a low sense of self-worth instilled during childhood. According to psychoanalyst Peter Hartocollis, editor of the book *Borderline Personality Disorders*,[9] the fact that he was born with a foot deformity was very influential. His lameness was treated by his powerful mother (his parents had separated before his birth) as a personal sin, and may have given rise to Byron's compulsive pursuit of love, prolific writing, radical social criticism and revolutionary activities. For the sake of his mother, he had to achieve a more perfect state, it is claimed. 'The same deformity that he experienced as a shameful "dark" secret made him feel entitled to be loved without having to love in return unless the other mirrored his own ideal,' writes Hartocollis in his article 'Lord Byron, his Mother, and Greece'.[10]

The impulsive, thrill-seeking behaviour and the feeling of entitlement certainly fits in well with modern concepts of narcissistic personalities. The man who effectively gave rise to the 'Byronic hero' himself exemplified some of the romantic characteristics that have lured and infuriated for two centuries since. There's a certain sense of self-loathing when Byron writes: 'Self-love for ever creeps out, like a snake, to sting anything which happens . . . to stumble on it.'[11]

Notes

[1] Jane Austen, *Pride and Prejudice*, Penguin Popular Classics, Chapter 3.

[2] Jane Austen, *Pride and Prejudice*, Penguin Popular Classics, Chapter 59.

[3] Steven Carter and Julia Sokol, *Help! I'm in love with a narcissist*, M Evans and Company Inc., New York, 2005.

[4] J Philippe Rushton, 'Mate Choice and Friendship in Twins: Evidence for Genetic Similarity', *Psychological Science*, vol. 16, Issue 7, July 2005, p. 555.

[5] Liliana Alvarez, 'Narcissism guides mate selection: Humans mate assortatively, as revealed by facial resemblance, following an

algorithm of "self seeking like"', *Evolutionary Psychology 2*, 2004, pp177–194.

6 Marion F Solomon, *Narcissism and Intimacy*, Norton, New York, 1989.

7 David M Buss, *The Evolution of Desire, Strategies of Human Mating*, Basic Books, New York, 1994.

8 Geoffrey Miller, *The Mating Mind: how sexual choice shaped the evolution of human nature*, William Heinemann, 2000.

9 Peter Hartocollis (ed), *Borderline Personality Disorders*, International Universities Press, 1977.

10 Peter Hartocollis, 'Lord Byron, his Mother, and Greece', *Canadian J. Psychoanal.*, vol. 6, 1998, pp15–34.

11 Byron's Letters and Journals, Ravenna Journal, vol. 8, entry for 11 January 1821, published in *The Works of Lord Byron. Letters and Journals*, Adamant Media Corporation, 2002.

4

WHEN MR RIGHT GOES WRONG

What it's like to suffer at the hands of a narcissist

Scratch a lover, and find a foe.

DOROTHY PARKER,
BALLADE OF A GREAT WEARINESS, 1926

Narcissism pervades every relationship to a degree. We all choose our partners, and make demands of them, partly to satisfy our own (possibly small) narcissistic tendencies. We all have an image of ourselves, which we may like or dislike, and in finding partners we are often attracted to those people who reflect back a nice image of ourselves – who magnify the bits we like, and compensate for the bits we don't like. As the British psychoanalyst Darian Leader has pointed out, some people enter a relationship for this purpose only. 'They need someone to reassure them, to tell them that the image fits. And this can lead to a comedy in relationships where one party will ask repeatedly for the other's approval. The other says "Yes, you look fine" and then expects the questions to stop, which, of course, they never do.'[1]

This reflecting back of each other is to some extent normal. But people who seek out partners solely for self-affirmation will inevitably make those demands throughout a relationship. The more deep-seated and hidden their insecurity about themselves, the more demands they will make of their partner. If your partner has narcissistic traits, that can be exhausting and difficult. If he has a narcissistic personality, it can be virtually impossible.

A recent study demonstrated how the demands a narcissist makes of someone equates to what they believe to be romantic attraction. Researchers from the University of Georgia and Chulalongkorn University in Bangkok found that even in a 'collectivist culture' like Thailand, where attributes such as being caring are valued far more than being ambitious or selfish, people who had been identified as having narcissistic traits were significantly more attracted to people who gave them admiration, supported the narcissist's views, and offered them the chance of personal advancement.[2] In other words, part of the attraction was that they knew they'd get something out of it.

Talking to people who have first-hand experience of a relationship with a narcissist, it's astounding how similar their descriptions of their feelings are. Cases in point are Claire, who tells her story here, and Nancy, who you will remember from the previous chapter. The narcissism these two women experienced was extreme. But men with narcissistic traits, rather than narcissistic personalities, can make you feel dreadful too. For people who come within its reach, extreme narcissism can be demeaning, imprisoning, and corrosive to any sense of self. Maybe what Claire and Nancy say here will ring a bell with you too. Like other people talking about their experiences in this book, Claire and Nancy lay themselves open to criticism when their words are put in black and white. Sometimes they sound like victims, sometimes stupid, callous or bitter. Sometimes you almost suspect that it's the partner of the narcissist who had a problem – and indeed, as we'll see later in the book, their own attitudes and behaviour may not have improved their situation. But we should read these accounts generously, remembering our own confusion and irrational behaviour when in love. When you talk in person to women like these, you realise that it's an amazing release for them to be able to talk about what they've gone through. They've steeled themselves to tell a story that secretly they'll always be ashamed of – because they've always feared that it's all their fault. And in person they don't come over as victims, or weak or embittered at all. They are just bearing a lot of scars.

Here, first of all, is Claire's story.

❤

For two years, in my early twenties, I had a relationship with a man named Mike. I fell for him because he was gregarious and charming. But he didn't just go out clubbing – he seemed to have depths too, and I thought I'd really hit the jackpot here. He told me about his childhood, which seemed awful – he had a father who had attempted suicide, and a mother who I thought was very controlling and cold. He was on a postgraduate course with me, and he always had to be the best. When things went wrong, and he wasn't the best any more, he turned against the whole thing, got into arguments with his tutor, and decided to leave. It was as if once his whole identity as the blue-eyed boy of the course had gone, he had to completely turn against the whole thing and blame everything on the course organisers. He said he was too good for them.

I knew he had attempted suicide as a teenager, and that somehow added to his mystique. He said that I was the one to save him, and I thought I was. Maybe you have to be a bit of a narcissist yourself to fall in love with a narcissist.

On the day of a mutual friend's wedding, he put a wardrobe in front of his bedroom door and threatened to kill himself. At the time it was incredibly upsetting – we were all waiting to go to the wedding, and we just didn't know what to do. Looking back I realise he didn't really want to die. It was all about making a point. He did it for effect, and he knew how fearful I was about it because of his family history. When I came home in the evening there would be no sign of him, and I wouldn't know where he'd gone. At 3 a.m. he might be sent home in a police car because he'd got into some sort of accident, or managed to get into a fight.

He thought the world revolved around him. If he was nice to me, it was because he wanted me to love him, and to make him feel important. But that would alternate with such nastiness. It was a deliberate sort of nastiness, designed to belittle you, and make you feel that you are nothing without him. I think, looking back, that it was because he was so insecure about himself. By being horrible to me, he was effectively saying: you're so worthless that no one else could love you. Only I could love you, and therefore you won't leave me.

Towards the end of our course (he came back in the end), I'd made up my mind that I was going back to London, and wouldn't live with him any more. I'd told Mike this, and he seemed okay about it. But then, on the last day of the course, out of the blue, he took an overdose. We had lunch, he left – said he was going home – and then in the evening I got a call from a friend who had found him comatose on the stairs, somewhere very prominent where he knew he'd be found. So what happened? I couldn't just leave him because he had nowhere to go, so I took him to London to live with me. He said I was the only one to help him, to save him. I was too scared to say no, because he had just tried to kill himself.

He had this curious detachment from other people's feelings. I suppose he was caring in the abstract – he made big gestures to make people feel good, like buying them presents, and talking about them all the time. But to be honest, I think people were sometimes wrong-footed by it all, because it didn't fit with how remote or rude he'd be most of the time. People didn't know what to make of him, and I think that actually made him incredibly isolated in the long-term. He didn't really have many close friends.

He seemed to have no appreciation of the way his behaviour was affecting me. I spent half my time distraught because I didn't know where he was, or because he was so unpredictable that my own life was becoming chaotic. And he used to say weird things like, if anything ever happened to me, he'd look after me and make sure I was all right. But then it happened – I had an ectopic pregnancy, and was very ill for weeks. And he was just horrible. He somehow made me feel it was all my fault, and just had no thought for how I was feeling. I just cried and cried, but it didn't seem to get through to him.

Not long after that, he started having an affair with a girl from work. I suspected something was going on, and a mutual friend confirmed it. I confronted Mike. You'd assume, wouldn't you, that a man confronted with evidence of having an affair would say either 'It's a fair cop, I'm off', or 'Let's try to work it out'? But neither of those seemed to enter Mike's head. His response was absolutely indignant. He said he was actually helping this woman because her partner was beating her up, and said it was very selfish of me to confront him. How dare I? And the weird thing was that he was so adamant that he was convincing. I almost believed what he was saying. After that, I didn't know where I was with him. Sometimes he would come home, sometimes he wouldn't. When he did come home, he would say how much he loved me, but the next day he would phone from work saying he wasn't coming home that night, and I wouldn't see him for three days.

I was thinking about getting an injunction. He wouldn't leave my flat, and I found it incredibly hard to say 'We're finished', because he made me feel so incredibly attached to him. He also threatened he'd kill himself if we split. We did finish in the end, after the only physical fight I've had in my life. I can't believe

I did it, but I remember punching him. I left the house so he could clear all his stuff, and get out. But even then, he made it difficult for me: he got out all the pictures of us together that he could find, and put them on the table waiting for me when I got home.

Once I was hooked on him, I couldn't get off – partly because I just thought it was wrong to abandon people who needed help. It was very difficult to walk away. Maybe I just wanted to be needed – maybe narcissists just prey on that.'

There are many strands to draw out here about how narcissists make you feel if you're in a relationship with them. Maybe you'll recognise some of the feelings yourself. Here are some of the main strands from Claire's story about the emotional turmoil you can go through if you're in a relationship with a narcissist – with further illustration from Nancy's story.

HOW A NARCISSIST MAKES YOU FEEL

Protective

I couldn't just leave him because he had nowhere to go.
Like Claire, those who are in relationships with narcissists often sense their vulnerability. Sometimes, amid their arrogance, narcissists will reveal their inner doubts in a surprising and emotionally affecting way. Their partner, having got into a relationship with someone who is dependent on them (even

though they may refuse to show it), feels responsible for the narcissist's welfare. This can be exacerbated because of the risk-taking, sometimes self-endangering, behaviour characteristics of narcissistic personalities. They need looking after.

When I asked Nancy why she didn't leave Roger, she said one of the reasons was sheer compassion. 'He has nowhere to go, and no friends or family. He doesn't have a job, he doesn't have anything. It makes me feel really guilty – if I left him, I'd have a fabulous life, but what on earth would he do?'

Unable to plan

I didn't know where I was with him. Sometimes he would come home, sometimes he wouldn't.

Narcissistic people sometimes lead very chaotic lives, and this can have a knock-on effect on those around them. It's all to do with that deep-rooted unpredictability – the thing that can make them attractive in the first place. It's fine when impulsive behaviour results in a bunch of flowers, but it's an entirely different matter when it results in staying out all night.

The psychoanalyst Michael Knight told me that the un-predictable behaviour of narcissists is very closely tied up with the reason they become narcissistic in the first place. When they were brought up, they didn't have the nurturing stability that can help them make sense of all the different, and sometimes frightening, emotions we experience as children. They are left with a fractured pattern of behaviour because their emotions are themselves fractured. Each circumstance sparks an emotion, and each emotion is responded to spontaneously, rather than being influenced by a central strong reference point of self – a still point that can help moderate extremes.

'The difficult bits in the way people relate has become very extreme – they aren't mixed up with each other in the way they should be,' he says. 'Each is dealt with separately and in a completely unpredictable way – so that you go from loving behaviour to contemptuous dismissal, which is actually how they [narcissists] feel about themselves. They pretend to be wonderful, but in reality they are something they can't bear to look at.'

Like Claire, Nancy told me that much of her life has been spent covering up for her partner's bad behaviour, or inventing elaborate stories to get out of arrangements that she knows will cause embarrassment or disaster. 'I feel I have to plan our lives incredibly intricately so that things don't go wrong, but that's incredibly difficult when Roger has no concept of the way his behaviour affects other people.'

In a state of fear

I was too scared to say no.

It's certainly not true of all people with narcissistic traits, but those with strong narcissistic tendencies can instil fear because of their unpredictability. There's always the risk of that sudden outbreak of rage. Those who have constructed a fiction or an image to support their idea of themselves can feel immensely threatened if that begins to be challenged, or its flaws start to become apparent. They can feel threatened by defeat. Like

Claire's partner Mike, they can feel threatened by anyone being better than them at anything. As Nancy says, it's like permanently walking on eggshells.

❤

If I left, I don't know what Roger would do. He's never hit me, and I've always sworn – and he knows this – that the moment he hits me I'm out. I often wish he would, because then that would solve it all. But sometimes I think he's capable of doing anything, even very violent things. And if I left, I worry about how the barriers might come down.

Daily life is one round of thinking 'How do I break this to him?' If I'm going to meet someone, or someone's coming round, or there's something we need to do, I have to consider when would be the right moment to tell him, what is the best way to couch the question. You have to consider and plan everything. I have to sit down and look at the diary every Monday and to plan the week ahead so that it's not going to upset Roger.

❤

Putting your life on hold

He was so unpredictable that my own life was becoming chaotic.

We've seen how Claire became unable to live her own life at all, so great was the time and energy she put into Mike. The same happened with Nancy. And the long-term effect of this can be that all career considerations and long-term planning for the future go by the board. A partner of a narcissist will often feel their life is completely on hold. It's something their friends will point out to them first – because dealing with the day-to-day realities of a chaotic life, it's often hard to get your head above water and see the bigger picture.

Nancy explains:

❤

It drives my friends mad that I won't leave him, I ignored my friends' advice for so long that it was years before I really noticed how weird my world was. Roger and I would go somewhere together, and we'd meet some people, and the next time I saw them on their own, they'd gee themselves up to say at the end of the evening, 'What are you doing with him?' But it's strange. Even after they'd said it, it didn't make me seriously consider breaking up – I rationalised it by thinking that they just don't get him. It didn't penetrate.

❤

Hooked

Once I was hooked on him, I couldn't get off.

Why, given all they are subjected to, do people like Claire stick with strongly narcissistic partners? The feelings induced in those who have relationships with narcissists are extremely complex, and can't be entirely separated from the feelings of love, or being in love. Yes, there is entrapment – a feeling that you have a duty of protection, a weird determination to finish the job you started, and a fear of what will happen if you leave.

But there's also something else – an addiction or dependence that has its root as much in the person living with the narcissist as with the narcissist themselves.

'Nothing else seems as exciting or as tangible as with Roger,' says Nancy:

There's something. I've looked on the internet chat rooms, and they are full of all these women who feel the same way: Why is it my fault? Why can't I leave?

I do love Roger, but in a different way to most 'normal' relationships. I think real love is what you do every day of the week, sitting down and talking about your worries and so on. Maybe you could describe it more as the 'in love' thing, but I think it's more than that. It's almost as if we have, to some extent, a survivors' bond. We've been through all these terrible things together and nobody else can truly understand, because they weren't there to ex-perience it. And, there's always been a strong feeling of waiting for my life to begin. If I could just make Roger happy and be a better wife, then everything would be okay. There's an addictive nature to the relationship. Maybe it's like compulsive gambling. If I just take one more chance on him, then this one will be the one that pays off.

I feel better when I'm not with him. I feel calm, because I'm no longer running on adrenaline. I'm not waiting for something dreadful to happen. I'm just being. But I still can't leave.

Self-doubt

The weird thing was that he was so adamant that he was so convincing. I almost believed what he was saying.

Fact and fantasy can be difficult to distinguish for those with strong narcissistic personalities. For those in their lives, like Claire, there's a knock-on effect. If the person whose life is interdependent with your own has a different idea of the truth, and if the conviction behind what they say is frightening in its force, your own sense of reality starts to spin. Most of us are subject to doubts when challenged – even narcissists. But narcissists have an ability to cover up challenge, to mentally wipe any alternative version of reality that might cause them to reconsider their own elaborately constructed vision of the world. The rest of us don't, and so it's us that end up reconsidering reality.

In the face of such a bludgeoning sense of alternative reality, it's not surprising that the partners of narcissists lose not only a sense of what is real, but also their self-confidence.

'Our relationship is a sort of crazy-making that scrambles your brain and manipulates you into believing things that aren't true,' says Nancy:

❤

Roger's truth is much stronger to him than anyone else's. He argues with me like a barrister. He spends £600 in a month on pay-per-view porn, yet when I pointed this out to him he said: 'You spend £300 on new shoes, so what's the difference?' He can't understand that it's not just the money. He doesn't think it's outrageous.

And there is a point where I almost believe him. I always feel I'm in the wrong. He got really pissed off when there was an article about my work refurbishing a country home – quite angry. It was almost like I'd done something terrible, like sleeping with someone. And that made me feel that maybe I should have considered doing the article more carefully, because I should have known it would have caused problems for him.

I think I've sacrificed my values for him. I've done things with him I would never have normally done otherwise. Roger got an idea into his head that he could only be fulfilled if he could have a sexual adventure, and we got into these sordid swinging clubs – which I really regret. I think he does this 'poor me' thing, saying his self-esteem is so low because women don't fancy him. And the other problem is he will be so nice to me if I'll do what he wants.

There's always an element of truth in what he says, and it makes me think the whole thing is true. I also think it's quite complex and insidious. Six months into our relationship, I wouldn't have gone to a swingers' club, but after six years you've lost your sense of self. That's what happens. You lose your sense of self. The relationship has left me so shattered, I'm not sure what's left of me.

❤

Humiliated

It was a deliberate sort of nastiness, designed to belittle you.

We know that narcissists are deeply competitive. They have to affirm their superiority. That involves sometimes making their partners feel worthless. That's certainly how Claire felt.

Nancy too has experienced this:

Roger's incredibly manipulative, so he constantly makes me believe I'm not good at what I do, be it work or at home. Everything makes him jealous. He doesn't believe I'm a good interior designer, and he tells me so. He doesn't believe I have any talent at all. He's also made me believe that I'm incredibly selfish, and that nobody really likes me, and everyone has a Machiavellian reason for hanging out with me. He makes me believe I'm dysfunctional.

Narcissistic personalities regard life as one long power struggle. That means that living with someone who is successful, and has normal social relationships with people, can be very difficult to deal with. It threatens their own fragile self-esteem. By acting hurtfully, they are looking to redress the balance by damaging their partner's sense of self-worth.

Sometimes narcissists don't just degrade the person they are supposed to love in words – they use their emotional power to force them to do things against their will. I've been told by a narcissistic man that he manipulated an orthodox Jewish girlfriend into buying pork sausages and cooking them for him. And as you'll have read above, Roger manoeuvred Nancy into attending a swingers' club – an experience he knew she would find totally humiliating.

Guilty

He somehow made me feel it was all my fault.

The 'somehow' is important. It defies all reason, but narcissists often seem to keep their hold on their partners by making them feel in some way responsible for their pain and bad behaviour. That certainly happened to Claire.

Nancy was persuaded to go to swingers' parties with Roger, even though she didn't want to. For him, it was all about power, about controlling her. But Nancy felt it was her fault – because she wasn't giving Roger everything he wanted sexually.

❤

There are all these appalling things he's done, but I feel it's my fault. It's largely down to Roger having made me feel everything I do is wrong. But also, after he's behaved badly or has been particularly horrible to me, he can be incredibly warm, loving and nice afterwards. And that makes me feel guilty too, because the juxtaposition with the awfulness makes the 'good' behaviour more powerful somehow.

❤

Angry

I can't believe I did it, but I remember punching him and punching him.

Anger isn't the sole prerogative of the narcissistic partner. Being with someone who constantly represses your sense of self, who puts your priorities below theirs, can be infuriating in the extreme. The pot is bound to boil over every now and again.

Powerless

I left the house so he could ... get out. But even then, he made it difficult for me.

Claire felt she was in a situation she was unable to control. This chimes with the experience of Nancy, who talked earlier about how she got worn down – how it became impossible to continue resisting the will of her partner. In the end, she felt she lost her sense of self.

❤

If you had firm boundaries in the face of a narcissist, the relationship wouldn't last. So you have to be flexible to maintain a relationship. The longer you stay together, the more you have to lose in ending the relationship, but when someone has isolated you from your friends, and you've been made to start to believe things that aren't true, it's much harder.

Also, I think one builds up a tolerance to extreme behaviour. For example, most people would scream and shout at their husband if they felt they'd been in some way unfaithful. But when Roger was involved with any number of girls, he was much saner and nicer to be around. So I kept quiet for a while for the sake of peace.

♥

Isolated

People didn't know what to make of him, and I think that actually made him incredibly isolated.

People with strong narcissistic tendencies don't have many friends – not real friends anyway. They are detached from other people's feelings, which means relationships with anyone except their partner tend to be based on superficialities. They also get jealous of other people's friends – other people's lives in fact.

The end result is that those having relationships with narcissists end up feeling isolated. They're being reserved for the special attention of their partner, and are expected to direct all their energies onto him, or her. Many people involved with a narcissist have the peculiar experience of their friends, and the life they used to know, drifting away from them, along with everything they formerly thought of as normality.

'Everyone else knew there was something wrong with him,' says Nancy:

♥

There's something about him that makes people feel a bit repelled. I haven't seen a friend for nine weeks. I haven't left the area around where we live. It's just so lonely. We can't have anyone round at Christmas because I know there's going to be a tantrum.

One year, he spent the whole of Christmas Day in the bath. It's just very, very lonely.

💜

Unacknowledged
He just had no thought for how I was feeling.

Lack of empathy can leave you feeling incredibly neglected. Claire's story about having an ectopic pregnancy has strong echoes with Nancy's tale of giving birth:

💜

When I was in labour, it was very difficult and very painful. Being nice to Roger wasn't the first thing on my mind and I said something like 'Fuck off, I hate you' at some stage, as many women giving birth do. But then he told me I wasn't trying hard enough and we'd all be there forever unless I tried harder. Even at the time, when everything was a blur, I couldn't quite believe it.

And months later, I presume because I'd been bad-tempered at some point during the labour, he said, 'I think you ruined the whole experience of having a child for me.' He could only see things from his perspective.

💜

Indispensable
He said that I was the one to save him, and I thought I was.

It's a common experience of women who are in relationships with narcissists to feel specially 'chosen' to help. Well, they are. Their partner relies on them to provide for them and to do everything emotionally for them – to supply them with self-esteem either by reflecting their positive points, or by making them feel good by acting as a footstool. That early romantic rush of feeling flattered to be the only one who can love someone properly, make them feel alive, help them be themselves, evolves into something parasitic. The feeling of being special changes into a feeling of being drawn upon.

Fascination

He seemed to have depths too, and I thought I'd really hit the jackpot here.

One of the strange things about narcissists is that they can exert an enduring fascination. As we've seen in Chapter 3, there are many possible reasons for this, but it's one of the reasons why narcissists are hard to let go of. Nancy has her own way of putting it:

♥

I really like him, and there's no one I'd rather discuss a complex issue with. You know how when you try to think about space and it's all too large and too much, and Roger's like that. He's like everyone else but more so.

Notes
[1] 'N is for narcissism: A–Z of Relationships', *The Times Body&Soul*, 29 October 2005.

2 Pornsawan Tanchotsrinon, Kakanang Maneesri and W Keith Campbell, 'Narcissism and romantic attraction: Evidence from a collectivistic culture', *Journal of Research in Personality*, October 2006.

5
A WORLD WITHOUT LOVE

What creates a narcissist?

We are not alone. To pretend self-sufficiency is to deny
a fundamental truth. Human beings can only affirm their
living by giving to others. We are reciprocal creatures. We
need attachment. We need to be reflected back through the
faces of others. Love is the most important experience of our
lives. It begins with childhood, it transfers to parenthood
and it ends somewhere beyond our comprehension.
Love is intrinsic.

CAMILA BATMANGHELIDJH[1]

We've established that narcissism is a personality trait, that it's more common in men, and that it's a destructive influence on relationships. But why does it happen?

Unfortunately, there's no simple answer about how narcissists are made. But true narcissism often has its roots in the way we're brought up, and the extent to which our parents develop emotional links with us as children. If we aren't nurtured as children, we can build destructive defence mechanisms around ourselves.

So this chapter will look at what we know and what we don't know about the way narcissistic personalities develop, and whether narcissists are born or made. Gaining some understanding of the origins of narcissism is important for those who have to deal with its consequences. If you can't change a narcissist, you can begin to understand them, and adapt your life to take account of their characteristics. Having asserted that most narcissists are men, I'll also be asking whether narcissism has something specifically to do with being male. Is traditional thinking on the way boys should be brought up contributing to the number of men showing narcissistic characteristics? Finally, I'll take a look at some of the biological factors that might also be contributing.

NATURE OR NURTURE?

Since the beginning of the twentieth century psychoanalysts have been explaining narcissistic traits in terms of our internal development since infancy. But our increasing understanding of the human genome in the past half-century has led to increasing speculation that personality traits that were previously thought the result solely of our upbringing are also the result of our genes. Studies have indicated that certain aspects of our personality are inherited. In fact, some researchers believe that genetic factors account for 50 per cent of the variation in many personality traits.

How much does this apply to narcissism? W John Livesley, a Canadian doctor specialising in personality disorders, published a paper in 1993, which concluded that narcissism could be largely inherited.[2] He did this by comparing the characteristics of identical and non-identical twins. Identical twins have an identical genetic structure, while non-identical twins have different genes. So if a trait is genetically influenced then it follows that identical twins will display similarities more than non-identical twins. If a trait is influenced more by the environment, you would expect identical and non-identical twins to be roughly similar. Livesley asked each twin to complete a questionnaire that assessed 18 types of personality disorder, including narcissistic personality disorder. Using sophisticated statistical analysis, he separated out the environmental and inherited elements of their answers, and concluded that of the 18 personality disorders, narcissism was the most genetically determined. He concluded not only that narcissistic personality disorder was partly inherited, but that 'normal' narcissistic traits were on the same continuum and were also partly inherited.

This certainly fits in with anecdotal evidence that narcissistic people often seem to have mothers or fathers who were also narcissistic. That's something we'll deal with more in a moment. The problem is that the interplay between our genes and our environment is a very complex one, particularly in the case of personality traits, which seem not to be determined by one or two genes, but by intricate combinations of many. We know that many genes are triggered by environmental factors – having the genes makes us susceptible, if you like, but it takes something in our upbringing or surroundings to fire them off and thereby for us to acquire a certain characteristic. And it gets more complicated. Scientists now know that the genes we are born with aren't set in stone – the way they work can be subtly altered according to our environment too (this is called epigenetics).

We still don't know exactly how all these factors interact in determining our personalities, though it's certain that our parents' personalities play an important part, if only in determining our susceptibilities.

So although Livesley's study is useful in establishing that narcissism might be at least in part determined by our genes, it doesn't really tell us how, or how much. What is clear, however, is that whatever your genetic structure and your inner susceptibility, your upbringing has a key role to play in determining your personality, and whether you will turn out to be a narcissistic type. And that's important, because it means that as both offspring and parents we can try to break some of the destructive patterns set up during childhood, and curtail the cycle of generation upon generation of parents creating generation upon generation of narcissists.

WHAT YOUR PARENTS DO

We saw in Chapter 1 how psychoanalysts developed their thinking on narcissism and its origins. Freud and his followers have generally believed that we were all born with an inbuilt primary narcissism. As infants, we are the centres of the universe, with those around us there only to cater for our needs. This sense of centrality breaks down as we grow and encounter the realities of life. We face the need to compromise and take into account the needs of others.

Dr Les Carter, a psychotherapist from Texas, has quite a unique take on this. In his book *Enough About You, Let's Talk About Me* he equates narcissism with the religious idea of original sin.[3] All of us have some traces of raw and rampant selfishness, he says, and this is evident from a child's earliest years. Toddlers' ranting and tantrums, he tells us, are not just a symptom of immaturity but of total self-absorption. They cannot see their needs and wants in the context of everyone else. Try persuading a toddler to share, or to see something from someone else's point of view in an argument.

This self-centredness, he says, is man's natural state. In fact, it's a reflection of what is known in Christian terms as original sin – the sin that Adam and Eve brought on every baby born because they had defied God and tasted the apple from the Tree of Knowledge. 'Whether you regard the Garden of Eden story as truth or fiction,' he writes, 'it's a contradiction of reality to deny that tendencies to unhealthy self-absorption are a fixed presence in each personality.' What most of us do, he adds, is grow out of that phase, and learn traits such as empathy and consideration for others.

Whatever you think of his religious slant, Carter neatly encapsulates the idea that narcissism is not the monstrous growth of selfishness, but the inability to shed natural and in-born selfishness. It's a slightly different angle on what Freud and his followers say about the 'primary' narcissism in all of us. Successive psychoanalysts have defined the process of growing out of this in-born self-centredness in different terms, but generally all of them see children growing up psychologically by overcoming a long series of barriers to the idealised and self-centred notions they have as babies and toddlers. The ideas, for example, that the world revolves around them, that they are at one with their mothers, that their parents are awesomely powerful, that they have the ability to do anything. Throughout our childhoods, we come up against challenges to all of these – and if they are overcome gradually, and with the understanding of our caregivers, we survive these challenges and move on, with our idea of the world subtly altered but our self-esteem intact. That's how we begin to live in a real world, a society inhabited by other people.

What happens, though, if you come up against those challenges in an uncaring environment? What happens if you don't feel love at the same time as all your childish, narcissistic perceptions are challenged? Well, first of all, the setbacks and disappointments encountered during this process would seem far worse. You'd feel challenged, insecure and unsure what to do. Rather than move on, knowing that you'll have support during this strange journey, you revert to more childish strategies for coping – for example, pretending that it's not happening, and that you really are the centre of the universe.

Second, you don't learn empathy. Child psychologists believe that only when infants have attention bestowed on them can they begin to learn about the value of love and attention to others generally. Researchers at the University of Washington have found that not only do infants learn new skills (such as tying shoes) by imitating caregivers, but they can learn feelings such as empathy by imitation too. Their experiments, using brain-scanning techniques, indicate that a specific part of the brain is activated during tasks where a student is imitating something from a teacher. The researchers believe this part of the brain may play a role in determining whether an action is being carried out by yourself or another person, and that by imitating we develop a sense of another person's perspective.[4]

On a simple level, it's a matter of learning by example. If children experience love and attention, they absorb the worth of both as human characteristics, and their in-born sense that their own needs come first begin to fade. Gradually they develop a sense of empathy. It's a process that continues throughout childhood, as a parent emotionally engages with their child – interacting, listening and discussing concerns rather than simply telling them what's right and wrong.

So if a parent doesn't spend time with a child, providing a

model for it to imitate, their sense of empathy may be slower to develop. The child also simply won't have a role model from which to absorb love and attention as human characteristics, or the benefits they can hold.

Third, and perhaps most importantly, your sense of self suffers. If you grow up in a family structure where your needs are inadequately addressed, you don't feel valued for who you are. From the earliest age, you might not get the attention and reassurance you need to give you a sense that it is safe to be yourself. As you grow, and need help, your needs seem to come second to other people – even to your caregiver – and you begin to feel isolated and unappreciated. Your sense of self-worth suffers badly, and you don't develop a genuine sense of confidence. Your caregivers have not given you enough grounds to believe that you are capable of successfully overcoming all the emotional barriers to come.

But you have to survive emotionally somehow. So you hide away your internal voice, and build a system of coping mechanisms around yourself. You stow away that aching sense of a real self undeveloped, because it is too hurtful to address, and surround yourself with defensive structures that create an artificial sense of being strong and capable.

This, psychoanalysts and psychiatrists believe, is what creates the characteristic traits of the narcissist. The self-defensive shell they construct around themselves explains the self-importance, the obsession with their image, the arrogance and the creation of a fantasy existence. But it conceals a deep neediness and vulnerability – which accounts for the need for admiration and adoration, the envy, and the lack of understanding of love and other people's needs. That's why it's wrong to say that true narcissists are in love with themselves, no matter how image-conscious they are. They were not given the means to love themselves, so the self-esteem they demonstrate is an elaborate sham – something they are usually unaware of. It's actually real self-love that they need.

It's very hard to look back on your childhood and see in it the roots of some of the problems you are now experiencing. And it's certainly not the case that narcissism only results from an abusive, cruel, or even a detached upbringing. Sometimes caregivers adore their children, but simply don't give them the genuine and empathetic attention they need to grow up. Writing in the *Sunday Times* in 2006, journalist Ariel Leve told movingly of her own upbringing, and asked whether her mother's narcissistic behaviour had made her so emotionally detached that she herself was a narcissist. 'Can you love if you've never been loved?' she asked. 'It depends on what you mean by loved.' Ariel's parents divorced two years after she was born, and throughout her childhood she worried about how her mother would handle things. She felt her role was to reassure her mum. A typical situation occurred when Ariel was eight and was told she needed glasses. Her mum became hysterical, thinking her daughter would go blind. Her mother's emotions and needs always took over. On the other hand, her mother almost canonised her.

'I'm not sure if I felt loved,' she wrote. 'Needed? Yes. Wanted? Yes. Cared for and cherished and adored? Yes. But loved? Love felt like a responsibility I didn't want.'

Now, as an adult, she says, putting other people's needs before her own doesn't come naturally. But she's concluded that real love is loving in a selfless way. And the problem with narcissists is that because they can't love, they need other people to do it for them. Even if that person is a child.

So there seems to be a continuum here. Narcissistic parents give rise to narcissistic offspring because their inability to engage emotionally with their children's needs leaves their offspring emotionally deprived too, and likely to build up the same defensive mechanisms. Many authors and psychoanalysts have recounted how severely narcissistic people find it very hard indeed for their children to be the centre of attention, and expect the world to revolve around them instead.

But Ariel's experiences show it's not a simple equation to draw up. We should certainly be wary of generalising that people with narcissistic tendencies will always be the product of un-caring, remote and self-centred parents. For all the different degrees of narcissism, there are different degrees of parental detachment and self-centredness that can explain them. There's no detailed research examining how narcissists are shaped, and what characteristics arise from what aspects of their upbringing – or indeed how much emotional deprivation it takes to have an effect on a child's personality. There is no simple relationship between, say, the amount of time a parent spends with a child, and how well-adjusted that child turns out to be to other people.

Some psychoanalysts have commented that people with narcissistic personalities sometimes come from broken families – they have been adopted, for example, or their parents separated. Others believe that narcissists tend to be much closer to a doting mother, and very distant from the father.

Some American commentators recommend very specific criteria by which people can find out whether their own parents were narcissists. Nina W Brown, in her book *Children of the Self Absorbed*, provides specific checklists for readers to 'identify a parental destructive narcissistic pattern'.[5] She asks readers to carefully consider their parents' behaviour in the past, and ask, for example, whether they turn every conversation to themselves, constantly demand attention, fish for compliments, fail to listen, use possessions without asking permission, find laughing at themselves hard, exaggerate and make demeaning comments about their children.

But the fact is that tracing the roots of narcissistic characteristics is not an exact science. Even those aware that they are narcissistic find it virtually impossible to trace this back to particular situations or events in their life – because their childhood, difficult as it may have been, is simply normal to them. It is impossible to view objectively because it shaped their personality, values and self-defence mechanisms. Many psychoanalysts have commented that some people who are confronting their narcissistic behaviour are convinced that they came from a caring background. At the same time, when they tell the psycho-analysts the facts about what happened to them during their childhood, it clearly cuts across this impression.

Bill, 40, is a man who is trying to come to terms with the fact that he is strongly narcissistic – his wife of four years has threatened to leave him several times. He's struggling to get to the root of his inability to give love, his unstoppable anger when he doesn't get his own way, and his urge to seek adoration and physical comfort from women:

♥

Where it all comes from, I can't tell you. I was adopted, and they say that adoption is a common trait in narcissists. To what extent it's causal, I don't know. The theory would be that because I was separated from my natural mother at six months, there was this gap. I often have this craving for skin contact, sometimes sexually, as if I'm craving the mother's breast. There's this theory that it's all about separation anxiety. And again, many narcissists are deeply insecure and that's how I feel. I have this overwhelming need for skin contact.

There is also this theory that real narcissism begins when children can't move on from their natural childhood narcissism. It's another of those contradictions. There's this image that narcissists are a colossus craving control, but I spend most of my time feeling like a small child. My behaviour is all about tantrums. I'm just like a toddler. I get so jealous, even of my own children. I have a son, Harvey, who is ten, who has a wonderful artistic ability.

And I resent the fact that he has at least one parent who is prepared to recognise and encourage that, and buy him books. The books I took to bed with me were an old sex manual and a history of warfare.

It's so difficult to talk about, because these are defence mechanisms that have been in place for 35 years. If part of the reason I behave as I do was being separated from my natural mother and then going into an adoptive family – then why didn't they recognise the attention I craved? And if I'm having to cope with something deep in me dictated even before I had consciousness, then the idea that it can be easily put right is ridiculous.

❤

BEING RAISED A BOY

With most psychoanalysts agreeing that the roots of narcissistic traits lie in a child's upbringing, they tend not to see narcissism in 'gendered' terms. In other words, they say its origins lie not in what sex you are, but in what your experiences are. From their own professional perspective, they are probably quite right.

But looking beyond a purely psychoanalytical perspective, and bringing in psychological, sociological and biological considerations, it's hard not to bring gender into the equation as well. There are certainly plenty of women narcissists around, but look at the evidence of people who talk about the problems they're having with narcissistic partners and they seem to be referring mainly to men. Most of the psychoanalytical accounts of narcissists are of men. And look at those classic narcissistic traits again: lack of empathy, arrogance, self-importance, an expectation of admiration. There is just something rather, well, male about them.

Michael Maccoby, in his fascinating book *The Productive Narcissist*, makes a strong case for the positive side of a narcissistic character – something we'll be looking at in more detail in Chapter 7.[6] He says that given the right circumstances, it's the narcissists of this world who make big moves and change things. They take risks and can have a vision, passion, a voraciousness for learning – all born of an inner insecurity – which drive them forward and ahead of others. At the same time, they have distinct weaknesses, which can bring the edifices they create tumbling around them: they don't listen, they are oversensitive to criticism, they can be paranoid and they get angry. Being control freaks, they are over-competitive, get isolated, exaggerate, lie and lack self-knowledge.

That paints a portrait – albeit caricatured – of male weaknesses rather than female ones. Female high-achievers may have some of those traits, but it is harder to imagine them becoming isolated because they refuse to listen to others. Why? Is it just a matter of nature – that when we talk about narcissism, we are simply talking about characteristics that are naturally male? Or are there some other mechanisms at work whereby society is creating narcissistic men? Or is there a difference between the male traits we see as narcissistic, and true narcissism?

With these questions in mind, it's interesting to relate the theories that narcissism has its roots in emotional deprivation during childhood (see above) to whether boys are brought up differently than girls. Much as they may love their offspring, and much as they may intend otherwise, the parents of boys tend to teach them to be tough, independent and cool. They don't encourage them to share their feelings, or express doubts and fears – at least, not as much as girls. They should be achievers ('He's going to be England captain, you wait'). And any boy who, over the age of five, is a 'mummy's boy' is bound to suffer terribly in the playground. So parents often discourage that sort of continued attachment too.

In some families tough-love can be quite obvious. Dr Sebastian Kraemer, a child and adolescent psychiatrist at the Whittington Hospital, London, believes society's emphasis on boys being independent has a major impact on their developing brains. He asserts that young boys are actually more emotionally and biologically vulnerable than girls at an early age, because they develop slower. That means that they actually need to be attentively cared for so that they can learn to self-regulate. If they are not left alone, but supported, loved and cared for in the pre-school years, then they become more adept at relationships, and less prone to being disruptive and aggressive. 'You hardwire in self-confidence that is not based on bluster, a self-confidence that is genuine and doesn't need to be constantly asserted,' he told the Royal College of Psychiatrists conference in July 2004. The archetypal Clint Eastwood-style tough guy – no name, no

relationships, no manners – would, he points out, in all likeli-
hood be a terrible father.

Interestingly, Kraemer backs up his theory by observing
that boys are more psychologically vulnerable to their parents
divorcing or their mother suffering from postnatal depression.
There's a physical and psychological need for attention in boys,
but anything that deprives them of this – whether it be the way
they are brought up, or deteriorating family circumstances –
seems to expose their vulnerability, with possibly lasting effects.
In the context of the way narcissism develops, this makes a lot
of sense. Being deprived of the TLC they need, they fall back
on primitive self-defence mechanisms – which makes them disruptive, attention-seeking and poor at maintaining relationships.

Kraemer is by no means alone in his belief about the
special vulnerability of boys to psychological harm from their
early years. Dr William Pollack, Associate Clinical Professor of
Psychiatry at Harvard University, has written a book called *Real
Boys: rescuing our sons from the myths of boyhood*. He points to
research showing that male infants are actually more emotionally
expressive than females, but that this changes as they get older.
Pollock believes this is because society, and with it parents,
demand that boys should stand on their own two feet. This
results in the boys developing a 'mask of masculinity' to hide
their shame, vulnerability and other feelings they cannot express
publicly.[7]

One of Pollock's colleagues at Harvard, psychologist Ronald
F Levant, has pulled together numerous studies about child and

gender development to demonstrate that in their first six months of life, boys are more emotionally expressive than girls.[8] He goes on to describe a social process by which these emotionally expressive young boys become taciturn, aggressive and – perhaps most importantly as far as narcissistic traits are concerned – unempathetic.

The process goes like this. First, mums work hard to manage their excitable and emotional boys. Second, at about a year, dads begin to influence their children's upbringing more, and tend to encourage activities and characteristics that are very 'male'. Third, both parents unconsciously tend to discourage boys from expressing vulnerable and caring emotions, such as sadness and fear. And finally, the child's friends and colleagues finish off the job – with boys playing games in large groups based around teamwork, toughness and competition, and girls playing games in small groups where they learn more about the emotional skills of empathy and self-awareness.

The process continues after that too, as the qualities of competitiveness and self-confidence are encouraged in a society that loves winners, whatever the cost. This will be dealt with in more detail in Chapter 6. But for the time being, let's just reflect on the fact that perhaps the way we're bringing up boys might mean many of them are a little more likely to develop problems which make them needy of love but at the same time uncon-ditioned to respond to love; untutored in the skill of empathy yet expert in competition; vulnerable but unable to understand or express that vulnerability.

If you were looking for a group that would be especially vulnerable to becoming narcissists because of the way they are nurtured, you'd have to say that boys would be prime candidates.

BEING BORN A BOY

Let's look at some other factors now, inherent in men from their birth, that might make those narcissistic characteristics a little more likely to manifest themselves. What about, in particular, the lack of empathy that seems to characterise narcissistic behaviour? It could well be defined as a male trait as much as a narcissistic trait. You'll hear it lobbed at men by a million women as they yell in the course of an argument: 'Don't you have any idea what I'm feeling? Why should I have to spell it out to you? If you cared, you'd understand.'

If lack of empathy is at the heart of narcissism, isn't it also at the heart of male nature? 'He never, ever, ever asks anything about me, or my interests, or why I love certain things – and believe me, I am an exuberant person always sharing ideas and questions and debates. But he isn't at all interested in anything that I cherish,' says a correspondent on an internet chat site for victims of narcissism. Couldn't she as easily have been one of the millions of women who write to agony aunts each day complaining about men's impenetrable skin?

Simon Baron Cohen, a psychology and psychiatry professor at Cambridge University (and the cousin of Ali G and Borat creator Sacha Baron Cohen) has conducted some fascinating research comparing the fundamental differences between the male and the female brain. In so doing, he has suggested that one of the key qualities of narcissism is also at the heart of male nature.

Baron Cohen investigated the idea that what we know as autism is in fact one extreme variation of normal male traits. Autism and its lesser versions, such as Asperger's Syndrome, are characterised by an inability to empathise with others. Baron Cohen's theory is that while the female brain is predominantly hard-wired for empathy, the male brain is predominantly hard-wired for understanding and building systems.[9] The extent to which a particular male or female brain will have these characteristics will vary according to the particular mix of hormones their brain was exposed to while in the womb. Generally, the more testosterone the male brain gets, the less empathetic it is, and the better it is at being systematic. At the extreme end of testosterone exposure lies what has become known as 'autistic spectrum' disorders. They could be called extreme maleness.

This has been demonstrated in recent research from Addenbrooke's Hospital, Cambridge led by Baron Cohen.[10] Researchers examined the hormone content of the amniotic fluid that foetuses were exposed to in the womb, and then followed those babies as they grew, examining their personality traits. They found the greater the amount of testosterone in the fluid, the less friendly the child grew up to be. 'While empathy may be influenced by postnatal experience, these results suggest that prenatal biology also plays an important role, mediated by androgen effects in the brain,' the researchers concluded.

Baron Cohen says that there are three common brain types – those where empathy is stronger than a tendency to be systematic (E brains, or female brains), those where the opposite applies (S brains, or male brains), and brains with a good balance between the two (B brains). Anecdotally, we would all probably make a guess that women would demonstrate more empathy than men. Women are far more likely to be found advising their friends on relationships while men are more likely to be perfecting the categories on their iPod playlists. Baron Cohen's research group at Cambridge has analysed the proportion of each sex with each of these profiles using personality question-naires, asking respondents to state how much they agree or disagree with statements like 'If I were buying a car, I would want to obtain specific information about its engine capacity' and 'I find it easy to carry on a conversation with someone I've just met'.

He found that for every ten men, six will have a male brain, two will have a balanced brain, and two will have a female brain. In contrast, for every ten women, four will have a female brain, four will have a balanced brain and two will have a male brain. In other words, half the men you meet will demonstrate a lack of empathy by pure dint of the hormones their brains were exposed to before birth.

He pulls together research to prove the point. There have been many experiments, for example, showing how from an early age, girls are much better at judging whether someone has been hurt, and picking up tones of voice and facial expressions. Baron Cohen points to an experiment where a single boy or girl was introduced to a new group of children who were already playing together. Girl newcomers tended to stand and watch for a while, and then gradually fitted in to the activity. This usually led to them being accepted in the group. Boy newcomers, however, were more likely to hijack the game, try to change it, and rather than fitting in would try to get everyone's attention. This 'look at me' approach was less successful.

Unlike Levant, Baron Cohen suspects this inability to empathise is at least in part in-built, not learned – and it's all to do with that prenatal testosterone exposure. His own studies have indicated that toddlers who had lower testosterone before birth had higher levels of eye contact with their caregivers – indicating more sociability and empathy.

There is other work that suggests men are narcissistic by nature as well as nurture. New research suggests that showing off, bragging and wanting to be the centre of attention goes back a long way in our societies. Anthropologists from Harvard University have investigated why, for thousands of years, men have gone out hunting, when it's a hit-and-miss affair that is far more dangerous than foraging and tending crops. They interviewed hunter-gatherer tribes in Tanzania and Paraguay, and separately asked men and women whether they'd rather live in a village of skilled hunters, or one full of inept idiots. Not surprisingly, the women said they'd prefer to live with the skilled hunters. But the men wanted to live alongside the morons, because that way they could show off their expert hunting skills to best advantage. They wanted to impress the ladies.

So how much is narcissism a natural phenomenon – a reflection of the way men simply are – and how much is it a phenomenon of our own making, a manifestation of the way we choose to parent?

The simple answer to a very complex question is that narcissists are made, not born. Yes, it's true that our genes partly determine whether our personalities will turn out to be narcissistic or not. Yes, it's true that many of the traits that are naturally male are also narcissistic traits. But does that add up to a full-blown narcissist – the type whose vulnerability and lack of empathy make them compulsive attention-seekers and fantasists with whom it is impossible to conduct a relationship of equals? Probably not.

It's certainly true that genetic and hormonal influences forge male personality traits that have much in common with the characteristic traits of narcissism – the attention-seeking, the lack of empathy, the competitiveness. But generally, if you assessed a male even with Asperger's Syndrome (a mild form of autism) who had a secure and well-supported upbringing against a checklist of truly narcissistic characteristics, they would be unlikely to score highly.

Let's go back to the checklists in Chapter 2. You'll remember the two sets of ten questions. It's quite possible to score quite high on the mild narcissistic traits in Checklist One – to

Were Shakespeare's tragic heroes narcissists?

Narcissism describes common human traits. Some would say it embraces the personality type of a large proportion of the world's population. So it is inevitable that any literature chronicling the full complexity of human nature will throw up narcissistic characters. No more so than works of tragedy.

The heroes of all Shakespeare's great tragedies show narcissistic traits. The origin of their tragedy is in their natural characteristics, because they find themselves in exactly the type of extreme situations that their personalities are most ill-equipped to deal with.

Hamlet is a non-productive narcissist trapped in a whirling cycle of self-reflection, unable to face the prospect of doing the wrong thing, and incapable of making the emotional leap into relationships.

Macbeth is a man obsessed with the idea of power and influence, who consciously tries to repress any natural human empathy to achieve his ends.

Othello is a man controlled by his own grandiosity, but under-mined by a deep insecurity about his worth that leaves him vulnerable to suspicion and jealousy. John Dexter, who directed the celebrated Laurence Olivier production of *Othello* at the National Theatre in 1966, said that Othello is a man too proud to think he could ever be capable of anything as base as jealousy. 'When he learns that he can be jealous, his character changes. The knowledge destroys him, and he goes berserk.'[11] There's a striking parallel here with narcissistic personality disorder – where those who have elaborately constructed a

fantastical world around themselves feel immensel~~
an obvious reality contradicts it.

But it is King Lear who arguably displays the most overtly narcissistic traits. He is so deluded by his own puffed-up image of himself that he cannot see himself or the world as they really are. He expects love from all around him, but is incapable of giving it himself until the closing moments of the play, when his pride has already wreaked havoc on his family and himself.

It isn't just his one great act of pride that marks him as a narcissist – making the dramatic gesture of dividing his land between his daughters, but only if they add to his sense of grandeur by declaring their love for him. It's the way he accepts the love of his one truly devoted daughter, Cordelia, not on its own terms, but as a means to add to his ego. It's the way he is thrown into a blind fury when his grandiose idea of himself is challenged by her honesty. And it's the way he persists in believing in a fantasy world, when all is falling around his ears: 'I am a man/More sinned against than sinning.'[12]

have narcissistic characteristics but not necessarily a narcissistic personality – but to score low on the characteristics of a narcissistic personality in Checklist Two. High scoring on Checklist One could easily be accounted for by normal human personality traits – particularly typically male traits. But scoring high on Checklist Two would suggest a genuinely narcissistic personality, and it is in this category where upbringing is likely to have

‑n crucial in creating characteristics that are problematic not only to the owner, but to most of those around them.

If we regard narcissism as a continuum on the scale of human characteristics, with 'nature's' genetic and male factors interplaying with 'nurture' influences from our upbringing, there's another question that raises itself. At what point does the 'nurturing' of narcissists stop? Is it just parental influences that encourage the development of narcissism, or are there also broader environmental influences that impact on us as we get older? That's what the next chapter addresses – whether, in fact, we're living in an age and society which not only reflects narcissism but encourages it.

Notes

[1] Camila Batmanghelidjh, *Shattered Lives, Children who live with courage and dignity*, JKP, London, Philadelphia, 2006.

[2] W John Livesley, 'Genetic and environmental contributions to dimensions of personality disorder', *American Journal of Psychiatry* 150, 1993, pp1826–31.

[3] Dr Les Carter, *Enough About You, Let's Talk About Me*, Josey Bass, San Francisco, 2005.

[4] 'A PET exploration of the neural mechanisms involved in reciprocal imitation', *Neuroimage 15 (1)*, January 2002, pp265–72.

[5] Nina W Brown, *Children of the Self Absorbed*, New Harbinger Publications Inc, Oakland CA, 2001.

[6] Michael Maccoby, *The Productive Narcissist*, Broadway Books, New York, 2003.

7 Dr William Pollack, *Real Boys: rescuing our sons from the myths of boyhood*, Random House, 1998.

8 Ronald F Levant, 'The New Psychology of Men', in *Professional Psychology: Research and Practice*, vol. 27, no. 3, 1996, pp259–65.

9 Simon Baron Cohen, *The Essential Difference: Men, Women and the Extreme Male Brain*, Penguin, 2004.

10 *Social Neuroscience*, vol. 1, no. 2, June 2006, pp135–48, 2006.

11 From programme notes to the National Theatre production by English critic Kenneth Tynan, 1966.

12 William Shakespeare, *King Lear*, Act III, Scene II.

6
GENERATION ME

Narcissism as a product of our culture

In the future everyone will be famous for fifteen minutes.
ANDY WARHOL, 1968

I'm bored with that line. I never use it anymore.
My new line is, 'In fifteen minutes everybody
will be famous.'
ANDY WARHOL, 1979

Star Listings International can offer you immortality. For just £25, you can have a star named after you in a constellation of your choice. Each star name package is carefully tailored to suit the occasion and is 'completely personalised'. Or how about having a frog named after you for 2,600 Euros? Or a water mite, a spider, a salamander? You name it, if it moves and no one's nabbed it yet, the company Biopat (www.biopat.de) will name it after you – for the right fee, of course.

Species and stars used to be named to commemorate their discoverer or famous people. But no more. Attaching your moniker to a heavenly body or an endangered arthropod is now within the grasp of anyone. We can impose our identity on the world without actually achieving anything, just by paying money. There are a million and one ways we can have our egotistical whims catered to every day. You can have a number plate with some obscure coded version of your name, you can put your face or logo on a postage stamp (the Royal Mail has launched Smartstamp software that enables you to create your own stamps), or have your photograph emblazoned on your luggage (Be a Bag, www.anyahindmarch.com). Little girls can have a doll made that looks identical to them (www.mytwinn .com), boys can incorporate their own images into a PlayStation game (www.eyetoy.com), and courting couples can send each other's names and love messages soaring across the sky trailing off the back of aeroplanes (www.flysigns.com).

Is there anything wrong with that? Not in itself. Asserting one's identity has long been hailed a positive value. In the 1960s, millions took Timothy Leary's advice to 'turn on, tune in, drop out' – to stop conforming to society's expectations and to do their own thing. In 1980s' Britain, individualism became a political prerogative, as Margaret Thatcher declared, 'You know, there's no such thing as society. There are individual men and women and there are families.' Capitalist societies, dependent on consumption and encouraging people to acquire personal wealth and status, are the ideal place for individualism. It's those who bask in the glory of competition and achievement who thrive in such an environment.

But at what point can we say that a society that prizes individualism becomes narcissistic? It's perhaps when that society takes on some of the psychological aspects of narcissism as defined by psychologists and psychoanalysts. One prominent commentator on American culture, Christopher Lasch, who died in 1994, said that the traits associated with narcissistic personalities appear in profusion in the everyday life of our age – for example, a dependence on the love of others, a sense of inner emptiness, boundless repressed rage, a fascination with celebrity, a fear of competition, and deteriorating relations between men and women. He saw a culture that had a sense only of self, not of others, and only of now, not posterity – very much mirroring the self-centred universe of narcissists who have no empathy for those around them and act impulsively with no thoughts of the consequences.[1]

So does our celebrity-obsessed, high-achievement society reflect the characteristics of narcissistic personalities? There's certainly an argument that the pressure is on to be a competitive attention-seeker. Being humble, honourable and a good loser are rarely cited today as qualities we should aspire to. Advertisements, sport, magazines and television encourage the view that being a winner, a high-achiever, is the only option. Reality television programmes like *The X Factor* and *Big Brother* centre on the belief that anyone can be a star, and magazines feed our fascination of being like celebrities. And yes, the body beautiful is always there before us, an object of desire constantly dangled before us on television, in magazines, and as the potential end product of a thousand and one potions, diets, cosmetics, surgical procedures and fitness programmes.

It's the 'Look at me' culture. As leading psychoanalyst Darian Leader says, 'If individualism is all about self-sufficiency, narcissism depends on other people. This is because we need other people to reflect our identity back to us.'[2] Narcissists cannot live without an admiring audience, and a society that doesn't just promote individualism but panders to our delusions of grandiosity sustains the illusion of our own self-importance.

Can it be that such a society is creating a new glut of narcissists constructing fantasy worlds about themselves? Christopher Lasch believed that this was what was happening in America in the late 1970s, and it could have been happening in the UK since the 1980s. Lasch pointed to the fact that whereas psychiatrists used to see people coming in with obsessive compulsive disorders and phobias, now they mostly saw narcissists. 'If these observations were to be taken seriously,' said Lasch, 'the upshot, it seemed to me, was not that American society was "sick" or that Americans were all candidates for a mental asylum but that normal people now displayed many of the same personality traits that appeared, in more extreme form, in pathological narcissism.'

There is logic to this. As we've seen in the previous chapter, our environment during upbringing has an important part to play in the way our personality develops, so our cultural environment may also support the development of narcissistic characteristics. Our development from children into adults who must interact with others requires the suppression of the over-whelming narcissistic tendencies we are born with. If that primary narcissism is indeed a natural state, it is all too easy for us to revert to that state if our conditioning environment – whether it be our parents or our society – encourages the idea of the all-important self, rather than the need to adjust to others to be part of a society.

EVERYONE'S A WINNER

In Britain over the past 30 years, high achievement, competitive-ness and individuality have all had strong economic and political associations. High material aspirations drive consumer booms. In its fascinating wellbeing studies of UK attitudes and happiness, the research organisation the Henley Centre has charted the way that Britons are increasingly competitive in what they own – always having an eye on their neighbours and relatives to see what car they have, what household gadgets they've bought, what clothes they are wearing. But it's also making them un-happy. The Henley Centre has found that while disposable income has grown by more than three-quarters in the UK since 1980, the number of people who are happy with their standard of living has declined.

This competitive unease applies to many aspects of our lives – sport is a prime example. The old attitude of 'It's not winning but how you play the game' has been superseded by 'Winning isn't everything – it's the only thing'. So schoolchildren are groomed into hardened winners in the hope of England finally beating the Aussies at cricket, winning some Olympic gold medals, and driving an economy that can compete with the emergent giants of India and China. We must be assertive about our potential and our achievements, out-psych the competition, visualise success, and be top dog by thinking top dog.

For many of us, this doesn't come easy. But for narcissists – showy, deeply competitive, loving the limelight – it's an environment where they are bound to thrive. As we positively condone narcissistic qualities, we make narcissists the centrepieces of our culture. They're superficially fun, sometimes bizarre, want to win, and are so keen to hog centre stage that they're made for entertaining us 24 hours a day (at a distance). Look at *Big Brother* – the reality television programme that has increasingly become a showcase for people not only with narcissistic traits, but with full-blown narcissistic personalities.

Every series of *Big Brother* has a psychologist analysing each move of the house residents, as their interactions and activities are painstakingly recorded for the nation to view. The housemates, who seem to be chosen for their exhibitionist tendencies, bask in the amplification of their every move. In the 2006 series, psychologist Geoffrey Beattie noted the residents' narcissism. 'The obvious narcissist was Nikki,' he said. 'She is an exhibitionist ... everything characterised by grandiose behaviour ... and drawing attention to herself.' But he also pointed to the characteristic vulnerability behind such narcissistic behaviour. 'They tend to be very sensitive to criticism and they tend to criticise back ... All this behaviour is a defence mechanism.'

Meanwhile, these are hard times for the humble. Shyness is simply no longer socially acceptable. The London Shyness Centre uses neurolinguistic programming, psychotherapy and hypnotherapy to try to cure people of their shyness. Its brochure says: 'Confident people with high self-esteem are able to pursue their dreams and goals, they feel worthy of their achievements. This can be you. Be everything you ever dreamed of being.' This isn't a one-off: there are now a dozen or so shyness clinics around the UK.

What if you don't want to achieve? What if you don't want to make an exhibition of yourself? What if you're simply shy by nature? Well, since 1980 you'll have been liable to receive a new diagnosis called 'social phobia', for which there are now drugs available. University of Sussex researchers published research in 2006 saying the fact that shyness is being made a disorder signifies that society is very uneasy with those who don't conform to the assertive standards of the twenty-first century. 'The increasing medicalisation of shyness suggests that bashful modesty and reserve are no longer so acceptable and that to succeed we must be vocal, assertive and capable of gregariously participating in social life,' said Dr Susie Scott, a sociologist at the University of Sussex.[3]

So narcissistic traits thrive. And, just possibly, people who wouldn't otherwise develop narcissistic traits do so through sheer pressure from culture and peers. And perhaps, just possibly, mild narcissistic traits become stronger narcissistic traits.

As Lasch says, culture does have an effect on personality, and 'every culture works out distinctive patterns of child rearing and socialisation, which have the effect of producing a distinctive personality type suited to the requirements of that culture.'[4]

The ability of a narcissistic culture to create narcissistic individuals may not be simply the result of different attitudes to children and their upbringing. The subtle grooming of personality may continue after early childhood. As children continue to grow, their peers and the society around them begin to influence their characters and world view. Urie Bronfenbrenner, a renowned American psychologist, believed that the development of the child and adolescent is determined by a complex interaction of their immediate environment such as family and school, and their larger cultural context. If nothing else, a culture will help determine the way parents bring up their children, and the sorts of values they instil in them. And, of course, narcissistic systems seem to be self-perpetuating. Narcissistic people often raise narcissistic children. Narcissistic people create narcissistic societies. And narcissistic societies encourage narcissistic people.

YOU CAN BE LIKE YOUR DREAMS

The talent-free contestants on the pop talent show *The X Factor* gather in the video pod after being rejected by Simon Cowell and his fellow judges. Most are in tears.

'It makes you feel you're wrong,' says one. 'Everything you've based your life on is wrong.'

'It's all I've wanted to do all my life,' says another of the rejected.

Seventeen-year-old Kylie walks in for her audition, encouraged by her adoring mother. 'I'm a star,' she says. 'I will be having a number one single, and a massive album which tops the charts. I live to perform,' she says.

The audition doesn't go well. None of the judges think that she has the personality or the voice to make it in the music business. But she and her mother refuse to accept it. 'I believe I've got it in me,' she says. 'I'm going to make the most of my dreams and I won't let them go.' Her parting shot in the video pod is a tearful: 'Simon, you w*****, I'll be somebody some day, you watch.'

Admirable pluck or delusional behaviour? The fact is that every series of *The X Factor* throws up hundreds of contestants who genuinely believe they can be the next Robbie Williams or Mariah Carey. It's hard to understand why they have such a strong belief in themselves and their ability given the sound coming from their mouths and the evidence of the mirror. This is not simply an example of British youth having a dream and working hard to achieve it. There's something intrinsically fantastical about the widespread delusion that anyone can be famous. It's not just that they're deluded about their own abilities. It's the fact that the only way they think they can 'be somebody' is to be famous. It's almost as if an expectation has arisen that we all have a right to be in an adoring limelight, regardless of what we do.

Like America, the UK has become a society obsessed with celebrity. If we weren't so overwhelmingly obsessive about celebrity, websites like Celebrity Skin and Bodily Fluids (www.blackpitchpress.com/celebrityskin/film.htm) could never exist. Celebrity Skin can sell you urine, skin cells, bacteria ('cultures that have either come in direct contact with a celebrity or are progeny of such bacteria') and 'fecal matter' of film and TV stars, music stars, literary figures and sporting heroes – US$33 buys you three cubic centimetres of Robert Downey Jr's poo.

So it's clearly deficient to be a nobody. If you can't be famous, then you have to pretend to be famous and hope no one will notice the difference. The phenomenal growth of magazines centred on gossip about soap actors, film stars and pop artists has given us a way into their lives – we know so much about them that we can imitate them. We can have our hair cut like them, buy clothes like them (in the process making said haircuts and clothes totally unfashionable), and have cosmetic surgery to make ourselves look like them. Try Googling Paris Hilton lookalikes and see how many you can find.

We can even star in our own soap operas. The company eDv, 'The Personal Motion Picture Company' (www.edv.uk.com) promises to make you a film about you and your family that will be 'simple, inspired and "fromage-free"'. An average motion picture about your family, scripted, filmed and edited by top film-makers from the BBC and the New York Film Academy, will cost you around £3,000. But hey, it could be the next *Meet the Fockers* . . .

Alternatively, the London company Ichikoo (www.ichikoo .com) invites you to 'Star in your own movie' – a film of your, or your loved one's, life compiled from childhood pictures and old cine and video film, all tastefully set to music and commentary.

'Narcissism is the inevitable conclusion to what we call the limelight culture: our obsession with celebrity, fame and self-aggrandisement,' according to Chris Sanderson of the trends agency The Future Laboratory. 'It's the result of that most selfish of decades, the 1990s, when we kidded ourselves it was all about karma and Donna Karan zen, when, in fact, it was about a desire for spending that made the 1980s look like the austerity years.'[5]

And then there is the internet, a medium seemingly designed specifically with our narcissistic tendencies in mind. We 'Google' ourselves to find out just how widely we are known, and feel a glow of satisfaction when there's evidence of others acknowledging our existence. Blogs started as web logs, mildly diverting diaries and random thoughts from those few who happened to have their own websites. Now, they have evolved into must-haves – run by everyone from Michael Moore to William Shatner to your mates at work. In 2005 it was reported that a blog was created every second, and by the time you read this it will be one every nanosecond. Blogs give you presence, a sense of importance and an outlet for your most profound or trivial thoughts. You can be somebody, and sense that all those millions of people out there are hanging on your every word – even though they're probably not.

And then there's Second Life – the online game where you are a character in a virtual world where virtually anything is possible. If there's anything about yourself you don't like, you can reinvent yourself into a glamorous avatar, project yourself in a way you would never dare to in real life, and build things around you as you'd like them. It's a metaphor for twenty-first-century attitudes. We're increasingly aware that we don't cut the mustard when it comes to growing expectations of wealth, beauty and happiness. But to compensate, we're given the means to create fantastical illusions of our lives and selves. Whether they're real or not seems to matter less and less.

Behind our fascination with projecting ourselves on the internet lies some complex psychological issues, which reflect the nature of narcissism itself. As the American sociologist and psychologist Sherry Turkle pointed out, our preoccupation with projecting ourselves to the rest of the world via computer perhaps betrays a deep insecurity about who we are. 'We search for ways to see ourselves,' says Turkle. 'The computer is a new mirror, the first psychological machine.'[6]

YOU'RE BEAUTIFUL

You'll remember that some commentators have drawn a distinction between somatic narcissists and cerebral narcissists. Somatic narcissists are the ones that conform most closely to popular notions of a narcissist. Obsessed with their bodies, they'll flaunt their breasts or their pecs, brag about their sexual conquests and be permanently conscious of what others think of their looks. If you go out clubbing on a Saturday night, at least half the people you will see conform loosely to that description. The trappings of somatic narcissism have become an acceptable social norm.

Men have been accusing women of narcissism of the somatic variety for centuries, and they have plenty of evidence to back up their case today. According to a study by market analysts Mintel, in 2006 the British spent one billion pounds on cosmetics – more than anywhere else in Europe, and 40 per cent more than five years before. The boom has been led by style icons such as model Kate Moss, who fronts advertisements for several brands.

But men today are far from the take-me-as-you-find-me specimens they were in the 1970s. Male vanity, once regarded as indicative of femininity, is now accepted – even applauded – in the most macho of environments. Reports in 2005 that England and Chelsea footballer Frank Lampard waxed his chest and armpits prompted a short wave of derision in the tabloid news-papers – until it became clear that virtually every other Premiership footballer was doing the same thing.

You only need to look at film producers' choice of actor to play James Bond to see how times have changed. In the 1960s, they chose a heavyweight former factory worker (Sean Connery) with tattoos and an unashamedly hirsute physique. In the 1990s, they chose a clothes horse with a pout in the form of Pierce Brosnan, and the latest incarnation, Daniel Craig, has the highly defined muscles of a gym bunny.

Writer Mark Simpson, who in 1994 invented the word 'metrosexual' to describe looks-obsessed modern men, said in 2006, 'The metrosexual isn't dead. He's just dead common' – so mainstream that he isn't even worthy of comment any more. A 2005 survey of 2,000 teenage males for *Sneak* magazine found that on average they looked in the mirror ten times a day. They spent an average of £24 a month on 'grooming products' and, the research claims, 72 per cent would like a makeover. Nine out of ten used hairstyling products, half used moisturisers and one in four said they would consider having cosmetic surgery.

There's a serious side to all this. Reports published in the *British Journal of Developmental Psychology* show that girls are worryingly influenced by stick-thin celebrities and makeover shows where women are supposedly transformed from ducklings to artificially enhanced swans. Girls as young as five are unhappy with their bodies and want to be slimmer.

So far, the evidence on boys' insecurity about their weight is less conclusive. But there are other worrying problems emerging. The charity DrugScope is concerned that an ever-growing obsession with the ideal body image is causing increasing numbers of boys to take anabolic steroids to help build and define their muscles. In its annual survey of drug trends published in September 2006, it found that steroid abuse had become a serious problem in at least 55 per cent of the towns it surveyed, with students and young professionals aged 16–25 using steroids for purely aesthetic reasons. DrugScope says men are as vulnerable as women to the pressure from idealised images of beauty and fitness. According to Jim McVeigh, a reader in substance-use epidemiology at Liverpool John Moores University, there are an estimated 10,000 users in the north-west of England alone.

HOW DID WE GET HERE?

The growth of consumerism has been one of the shaping forces of a narcissistic culture. But there are others. Christopher Lasch believes that people lost hope of ever changing anything that really mattered after the political turmoil of the 1960s, so they turned inwards to live for themselves and the moment instead. Their lives became so cosseted and banal that people simply started looking for kicks. As Jimmy Porter said in John Osborne's seminal 1960s play *Look Back in Anger*: 'There aren't any good, brave causes left.'

Some sociologists believe that in a 'post-modern' age which reacts against a totally ordered and fixed view of the world, it is extremely hard for any of us to find easy ways to judge ourselves. Because of this, all sorts of new standards are coming into play to help us see how we compare to others. No longer (quite rightly) can we rank one another on the basis of race or class – something in the past that provided a convenient if artificial gauge of 'where we stood'. So we have had to devise other ways of judging. One way is through the appearance of our bodies – our weight and our appearance have become indicators of our confidence and moral control. If we weigh nine stone as opposed to twelve stone, it's a visual display of restraint. Equally, if we have finely honed muscles as opposed to a beer belly, it's a visual illustration of discipline. Our obsession with bodily appearance may be tied up with our attempts to position ourselves in a society where rankings are otherwise increasingly difficult to see.

The way in which we personally acclimatise to a culture's outlook may be subtle, but we all get drawn in. And, unfortunately, when it comes to the more narcissistic elements of our culture, our acclimatisation doesn't make us any happier. In fact, it's one of the ways that narcissism is ruining our lives. It pulls us into a world of constant concerns about our image, of comparing ourselves with other people, of insecurity under the guise of self-confidence. Our pursuit of self-fulfillment, of a place in the world, is ironically dooming us all to be permanently looking over our shoulders, wondering whether we are good enough to make it – something that the psychologist Oliver James has also drawn attention to in his book *Affluenza*.

Who can blame us? Our increasingly narcissistic ways are a mark of our humanity – our vulnerability and basic survival instincts. Can we blame young people for adopting increasingly narcissistic characteristics if it helps them fit in? Just as children are extremely vulnerable to the omissions of their caregivers, so as they grow into adults they continue to be vulnerable to the norms established in a culture.

This does not necessarily make them narcissistic. As we've seen, it's largely our early childhood experiences that seem to determine whether people go on to have predominantly narcissistic personalities. But our personalities are malleable to some extent throughout our lives. This is now being acknowledged by neuroscientists, who believe that as the human lifespan extends, so our personalities will increasingly be subject to substantial change during the course of a lifetime.

The fact is that after the genetic hand gifted to us at birth, we are all basically the product of our interaction with the world and other people. Who we are and how we feel are aspects forged primarily by our relationship with our mother, our other caregivers, our siblings, our friends and those with whom we fall in love. But who we are is also determined by our relationship with the world, our immediate environment, our society, our culture and our God too. We cannot escape them, and whether the experiences of those relationships are good or bad, they make us what we are. Living in a narcissistic culture is not an insignificant influence.

If you are having a relationship with a narcissistic person, our culture could be one of many influences that have made him or her who they are. It might have allowed them to have assumed a cloak of normality more easily – narcissists can be camouflaged against the background of a society equally ill at ease with itself. This is perhaps one of the reasons why people who have relationships with narcissists only begin to realise how problematic their characteristics are once the relationship is well underway.

Notes

[1] Christopher Lasch, The *Culture of Narcissism: American Life in an Age of Diminishing Expectations*, W W Norton & Company, New York, 1979.

[2] Darian Leader, 'Learn to love your image: N is for Narcissism', *The Times Body&Soul*, 29 October 2005.

[3] Dr Susie Scott, *The Times Body&Soul*, 8 April 2006.

[4] Christopher Lasch, *The Culture of Narcissism: American Life in an Age of Diminishing Expectations*, W W Norton, London, 1979, chapter 2, p. 3.

[5] Chris Sanderson quoted in 'Look at Me!', *Sunday Times*, 18 December 2005.

[6] Sherry Turkle, *The Second Self: computers and the human spirit*, MIT Press, 2005, chapter 9.

7
I'M A CELEBRITY NARCISSIST

Why narcissism helps people get places

Well, there's good news and bad news. The bad news is that Neil will be taking over both branches, and some of you will lose your jobs. Those of you who are kept on will have to relocate to Swindon, if you want to stay ... I know, gutting. On a more positive note, the good news is, I've been promoted, so ... every cloud. You're still thinking about the bad news, aren't you?

RICKY GERVAIS AS DAVID BRENT,
THE OFFICE, BBC TELEVISION

One of the reasons that narcissism is so 'in your face' today is that there are a lot of narcissists in positions of power, influence or public prominence. Some true narcissists fail miserably to do anything, paralysed by their insecurities. But others rapidly assume major roles. Why?

Well, it's not necessarily that narcissists project themselves as good employees – their unpredictability and irrationality emerge too obviously for that to be the case. But they are the sort of people who, given the right circumstances, can doggedly work their way to where they want, regardless of what anyone else thinks. They have a glorious image of themselves to fulfil. And their lack of empathy can be a positive boon when it comes to making tough business decisions.

Here's Daniel, a 36-year-old former director of a film production company who now recognises he may have a narcissistic personality. He looks back at his days in various positions with film companies, and realises that so much of what he did had less to do with the best business decision, and more to do with self-gratification.

❤

There have been three occasions where I've moved into senior positions and the first thing I've done is completely restructure departments. At the time, when I presented the papers to my superiors proposing the changes, and even as I explained to them the logic of these changes, I was convinced it was the correct thing to do. But now, looking back, I actually think I did it because I enjoyed making people redundant. And the reason I enjoyed it was because it made me the centre of attention. By making decisions that affected people professionally they were in my thrall. It was all to do with power. I wasn't aware of it at the time, and I've shied away from the fact that I enjoyed the process, convincing myself that it was for the best. But now I see it for what it was. On each occasion, I enjoyed the drama that I had created.

❤

Daniel's personality may have got him a long way, but it didn't last. He now describes his career as in 'freefall'. In the end, no one else could work with his anger, his unpredictability. In fact, he realises, virtually every person he worked with hated him. So he was pushed out, and hasn't been able to rally himself since. He's entirely financially supported by his wife, Gilly.

❤

'I haven't been able to work since I've been trying to control my narcissistic behaviour. Before, it was like white water rafting, and everything gave you a buzz. But the idea that I have to be in control of myself now – well, it's almost unthinkable. It's the difference between taking control of other people, which I want to do, and control of myself, which I can't.

❤

Daniel is far from a success story. He had such strong narcissistic traits that the world caved in around his ears. People like him appear to be high-flyers for a while, but, in the end, their inner need to be the centre of attention at all costs cuts across the larger objectives of their employers.

However, there is another side to this. The psychoanalyst and business consultant Michael Maccoby says that we should make sure we view 'narcissistic' as one of several personality types, rather than a damning judgement on people's selfish qualities. If we do so, he says, it becomes apparent that narcissists are exactly the type that reach the top despite all the obstacles in their way. A true narcissist, he says, is someone who doesn't listen to anyone else when he believes in doing something, and who has a precise vision of how things should be. On this basis, Maccoby is able to compile a long list of people who have reached the top on the basis of a narcissistic personality type.

Here are a few of them: Steve Jobs, Oprah Winfrey, Abraham Lincoln, Bill Gates, Franklin Delano Roosevelt, Napoleon Bonaparte, Charles de Gaulle, Mao Tse-tung, Leonardo da Vinci, John D Rockefeller, Duke Ellington, Bill Clinton, Richard Nixon, Ronald Reagan, Richard Branson, Frank Lloyd Wright, Camille Paglia, Pablo Picasso, Coco Chanel, Helena Rubenstein, Orson Welles, Francis Ford Coppola, Stanley Kubrick, Marlon Brando, Richard Wagner, Miles Davis, Louis Armstrong, Winston Churchill, Marcel Proust, James Joyce, Ernest Hemingway, Vincent Van Gogh, Henry Ford.

These are what Maccoby calls 'productive narcissists'. That is, the narcissists who change our world are the ones who have the charisma, drive and communication skills to catch a wave of feeling at the time, then to get others to buy into their vision and help them make it a reality. The converse of this is the unproductive narcissist – someone like Daniel, or Ali's boyfriend Sebastian (see Chapter 3), who spent all his days strumming his guitar rather than trying to achieve something.

Unproductive narcissists retreat into their own world, become increasingly isolated, and in their delusion blame others for their lack of achievement and loneliness. Productive narcissists, on the other hand, end up chief executive of a multi-national corporation. Their faults are much the same: they can be irrational, prone to anger and totally lacking in empathy. Productive narcissists still tend to be over-sensitive to criticism, over-competitive, isolated, and grandiose. They tend to exaggerate and not to listen to people – like all narcissists. But what draws them out is that they have a sense of freedom to do whatever they want rather than feeling constantly constrained by circumstances. They are active rather than passive, and have a sense of purpose that continually drives them forwards. In this respect, their grandiosity is a positive – they have an image of themselves and their world that has to be made reality, whatever the cost. And though their lack of empathy for other people is in some respects a problem – narcissists are not great 'people people' or team-builders – that same romantic charisma that makes so many male narcissists attractive to women can also help draw people into their vision, and produce a cohort of disciples who will pursue the dream for all its worth.

In truth, narcissistic high-achievers in business or celebrity or the arts will have many of the same problems in their daily lives and relationships as narcissists who sit in their rooms all day. As Christopher Lasch says, narcissists come to the attention of psychiatrists for many of the same reasons that they rise to positions of prominence in business, politics and the media. Being bad at empathy makes them good at business, but bad at meaningful relationships. In bureaucratic institutions, which put a premium on the manipulation of relations, and discourage the formation of deep personal attachments, narcissistic traits can be a positive advantage. At the same time, says Lasch, they provide the narcissist with the approval he or she needs to validate their self-esteem.

What makes the crucial difference then? What determines whether a narcissist will be non-productive, or an up-and-at-'em full-blown force in society? It seems to be something to do with the exact balance of traits in the personality – whether the drive towards a dream outweighs the isolating elements of the same personality. As we'll see, there can be quite a fine line between narcissists who perform badly in the workplace because of their traits, and those who achieve outrageous success because of them. It may be that sheer will to win, and the charisma factor, are the difference.

The traditional image of the narcissist, summed up in the myth of Narcissus, is of someone so self-absorbed in their own image that they cannot tear themselves away from the mirror. The difference with narcissists who make it big in the world is that they cannot see an image of themselves they can be happy with unless they go out there and create it.

NARCISSISTS IN BUSINESS

Having got this far in the book, you've probably spotted several people in your life who you think are narcissists. Some will no doubt be work colleagues. It's remarkable what an impact the people who you work with can have on you – after all, many of us spend one third of our lives working before retirement. And narcissists are particularly likely to make their presence felt. You can't ignore them, because they don't want you to.

They're the people who seem to have a bulletproof belief in their own abilities, yet react horribly if there's even the faintest hint of criticism. They're not easy to work with because they aren't keen on helping others, and find it hard to join in the fun in anything but an attention-seeking way. Many will make a big splash when they arrive in a company – they'll be so full of themselves, so energetic and have such big plans that everyone will believe the publicity. For a while. But because of their innate inability to see beyond their immediate needs, most are doomed to be low to middle achievers. If you've ever watched an episode of *The Office*, you'll know, in David Brent, what a true narcissist at work looks like.

Timothy Judge, a University of Florida management professor, authored a paper published in the *Journal of Applied Psychology*[1] revealing that though narcissists constantly rate themselves well on leadership and job skills, their rating from supervisors and work colleagues is consistently lower. Judge and his colleagues surveyed 139 business administration students, and 143 lifeguards (yes, lifeguards) to see how they rated on narcissistic traits. Then they surveyed them and their work colleagues about how they did at work. They found that narcissists just didn't know their limitations. Judge concluded that this will keep them from trying to develop skills that will help them improve, or make their organisation work more effectively. He says that because narcissists lack empathy and have self-serving motives, they are less likely to contribute to a good office atmosphere, and more likely to become aggressive or undermine other colleagues if they think they are doing better than them.

Sounds as if narcissists are a disaster in a working environment, doesn't it? Well, they usually are in terms of working with other people. Narcissists like David Brent are always found out. But the fact remains that some of the highest flyers in the world of business have narcissistic tendencies. How do they manage it, in the face of everything that Judge and his colleagues found? What makes the difference between a David Brent and a Richard Branson?

Well, it seems that rather than working with people and therefore trying to engage with the people skills they patently lack, some narcissists simply manage to sidestep the whole process of working 'with' people by making themselves leaders from the very start. They don't fit in, because they can't. Instead, they pull everyone else behind them through the sheer power of their personality and vision.

It's interesting to note that experts in psychology and business also point to a number of other common factors that many big achievers have, and which are also common to narcissists. Impulsive behaviour is one – it doesn't necessarily help business leaders in getting to the top, it just seems to be something they all have a tendency to. Making snap decisions – whether it be to invest massively in something, or sack someone, certainly keeps employees on their toes. It's got something to do with that narcissistic yearning for excitement – if there isn't enough drama around, they will create it.

Another characteristic of high achievers and narcissists is charisma – not necessarily charm or likeability, but a certain something that makes them compelling to others. Some business psychologists have also spotted that deprivation in early life is a common factor of big entrepreneurs – it leads them to want more control over the world, and to do what it takes to achieve that.

Manfred Kets de Vries, a psychoanalyst and world authority on leadership skills, believes that many of the world's top business chief executives achieve great things because they are trying to compensate for the blows to self-esteem received from parents in childhood. This, he believes, can be the result of parents being too indulgent, as well as too distant, and he points to the number of narcissistic leaders who have been very remote from their fathers, but had their ego fed by an indulgent mother. Such indulgence can contribute to narcissistic injury because it inhibits a child from developing a coherent view of the world and a proportionate sense of their own abilities.

People with narcissistic injuries, he says, have a hunger for external affirmation to combat their low sense of self-worth. 'In my work with leaders, I have found that CEOs generally have no idea that narcissistic wounds underlie their behaviour,' says Kets de Vries, who is Clinical Professor of Management and Leadership at the European Institute of Business Administration.[2] Yet they succeed through being able to get people to buy into their ambitions, their personal drama, their dreams. They do it by a combination of passionate communication, inherent charisma, and turning on the charm. This makes sense – narcissists need to be able to charm people, to get them on their side, to be able to sense that admiration coming back. If they do it well, and get the adulation they think they deserve, it motivates them to get on with it and succeed and charm some more.

For all its bad press, narcissism can drive achievement. Without it, as we'll see in the following pages, history could have been very different.

NARCISSISTS LEADING THEIR COUNTRY

Anyone who achieves a position of power – who reaches the top of the pile in politics, government or the military – requires an extraordinary amount of drive. The evidence suggests that narcissistic traits have figured strongly in those who have led us and left their imprint on the world throughout history.

Name a dictator or a great military leader who hasn't been obsessed with their appearance. We know about Hitler's and

Mussolini's obsession with the best-designed, best-tailored uniforms. But Winston Churchill? He was nothing if not image-conscious – with his trademark cigar, V-sign and a red velvet siren suit made for him by a Savile Row tailor. Nelson? A brilliant self-publicist who made sure that every detail of his victories was relayed home. Wearing his ceremonial top coat, complete with glimmering medals indicating his past triumphs, was his downfall at the Battle of Trafalgar, when a French sniper picked him out easily on the deck of his ship *The Victory*, and fired a musket ball through his shoulder.

Great leaders' instinctive awareness of the image they project to the world may be a symptom of the same inner insecurities that drove them to reach the top in the first place. Some psychologists and other commentators say that this inner vulnerability is so great that we can speculate that the majority of men and women who have imposed their image on the world actually had personality disorders. Dr Thomas Stuttaford, writing in *The Times*, has said that the Duke of Wellington (who was a bit of a fashionista himself, his name immortalised in a boot which he had made according to exact instructions by his shoemaker) may have had a schizoid personality disorder. He says there is evidence that Wellington was indifferent to the praise or condemnation of others, aloof, cold and emotionally detached.[3]

In modern politics and warfare, we've seen some pretty horrible examples of leaders with personality disorders imposing their own sense of order onto the world. One example is Slobodan Milosevic, the Serbian leader who became the first

European head of state to be prosecuted for genocide, before he died at the age of 64 in 2006. He presided over mass murder in south-eastern Europe during the 1990s, and 'ethnically cleansed' more than 800,000 Albanians from their homes in Kosovo. When CIA psychiatrists profiled the leader during this time, they concluded that he had 'a malignant narcissistic personality . . . strongly self-centred, vain and full of self-love.'[4]

When you look at the facts surrounding his life and person-ality, Milosevic falls easily into the category of someone with narcissistic personality disorder. His parents separated when he was young. He achieved power by mesmerising people with his extravagant promises and rhetoric. He was unpredictable, and his grand plan for Serbia turned out to be complete fantasy. The former US ambassador in Belgrade is reported to have said of him: 'Milosevic can utter the most egregious falsehoods with the appearance of the utmost sincerity. He is a Machiavellian character for whom truth has no inherent value of its own.'

According to his *Guardian* obituary, he was a leader who 'won most of the battles and lost all the wars' – constantly living for the moment, for the thrill, for the attention, but with no regard for the long-term or how his actions were likely to affect others.

That is a narcissistic leader at his worst. But there are plenty of more positive accounts of leaders whose narcissism led them forward to change the world – ruthlessly, yes, but history has looked more kindly on them. Take Nelson, Wellington and Churchill. Or Alexander the Great. Alexander was hardly a peacemaker, but Kets de Vries makes a strong case for him as a man who changed the world largely as a result of constructively channelled narcissism. 'He had to continuously prove to himself in his "inner theatre" that he could conquer these lands and so had an enormous restlessness,' says Kets de Vries.[5] Or how about that great American social and political reformer Abraham Lincoln, who has been described as 'a narcissist who rejected the social demands in favour of his own vision, one that wasn't reinforced or encouraged by his peers'.[6]

Narcissists are at the forefront of human history. The traits that took them there may be destructive in many circumstances, but they have created the world as we know it, for good or ill.

NARCISSISTS IN THE CREATIVE ARTS

On a superficial level, creative people, and particularly artists, are prime candidates for being fingered as narcissists. Several of the people who told their stories to me have either worked in the arts, or are interested in the arts. This isn't entirely surprising. Creative people need to think out of the box a little, to cast new light on old things by being out of the ordinary and unpredictable. In the case of performing artists, perhaps all artists, there's a requirement to be a bit of an attention-seeker, to attract all eyes by the drama you are creating, whether that be on paper, canvas, stage or cinema screen. It's connected with that charisma factor – people can't stop looking at you. In that respect, artistic endeavour can be very attractive to narcissists. It gives them an outlet for their need to literally create drama. And fair enough, their attention-seeking can be amusing, moving, revealing or life-enhancing in an artistic context. Many of the best and most popular actors in the world have achieved the heights they did because of their essentially narcissistic tendencies: think Brando, Gielgud, Dean, Valentino, Welles. Glorious and gloriously self-conscious all.

But we have to be careful about taking generalisations about narcissism too far in the artistic world. Visual art, in particular, might superficially appear to be highly narcissistic. How many self-portraits, for example, did Rembrandt, Edvard Munch and Pablo Picasso paint? What about artists' obsessional interest in their own bodies? British sculptor Anthony Gormley has cast his own image thousands of time and uses his own body fluids to draw with. And Marc Quinn is best known for a sculpture of his head he created from nine pints of his own blood.[7]

Or what about artists' tendency to parade every detail of their personal life in front of the public? British artist Tracey Emin, for example, somehow managed to scandalise the nation by exhibiting her bed sheets and bedroom debris at the Tate.[8] Her works have been described as 'obsessively confessional'.

But despite the appearance of attention-seeking in such artists, it's a different kind of 'look at me' than that caused by the inner vulnerabilities of true narcissists. Rembrandt, Munch et al. didn't necessarily paint themselves because they had narcissistic personalities, but because they were there as models and cheap. Perhaps most importantly, they did it because looking into your own eyes is what artists have to do. Their creative endeavour is all about putting everything they are into their work, about squeezing out every ounce of their perceptions about themselves and the world around them, and transferring them into the things they create. Once it has been put into their creation, it has gone. Unlike true narcissists, artists want to be judged on their work, not on their own drama or glory. It's what the viewer or reader makes of the piece of art – not what they make of them – that is important.

So narcissists may be drawn to the trappings of artistic endeavour, expecting personal admiration to be reflected back from what they have created. But a real artist doesn't expect anything back.

CELEBRITY NARCISSISTS

All that you have read above about the way narcissistic qualities can provide the drive and dream to reach the top in politics, statesmanship and business also applies when it comes to those who get into the public eye in other ways: the people who become actors, pop stars, television hosts, comedians, or even the full-time 'celebrity'. These are the people who, unlike *The X Factor* failures, actually do have a bit of talent, and enough charm and inner will to take them where their fantasies direct them.

Programmes like *I'm a Celebrity, Get Me Out of Here!*, *Celebrity Love Island* and *Celebrity Big Brother* demonstrate the prevalence of celebrity narcissism. The shows are concocted around the assumption that if you put a dozen narcissistic types together you get a lot of competition for the limelight, a lot of anxiety about how others will perceive them, a lot of simmering jealousies, a lot of unpredictable behaviour, and some of the celebrities' delusions about their world being shown up for all to see. Occasionally those delusions are systematically dismantled. The action, and the entertainment, depends on those classic narcissistic tendencies – grandiosity, jealousy and an inability to see the world from other people's perspectives.

The 2007 series of *Celebrity Big Brother* was clouded by a row over whether some of the contestants had been racist or not to Bollywood star Shilpa Shetty. One of the participants involved in the controversy – model Danielle Lloyd – uttered some words during the event that summed up the eternal discontent in narcissists' drive for thrills and achievement. 'I want something to happen all the time ... but then when it happens, I don't like it.'[9]

But is it simply that all people who reach the top in celebrity circles have a natural overload of narcissistic traits? Or is there something about the world of the celebrity that actually creates narcissistic tendencies? In the previous chapter, we looked at the complex relationship between a person's environment and the personality traits they display. It doesn't seem simply that narcissistic tendencies are determined by the way your caregivers treated you. The environment and culture you were brought up in is also influential – if not in conditioning totally narcissistic personalities, then at least in exacerbating existing narcissistic tendencies. Could it be that the rarified air that celebrities come to breathe turns them into vain monsters?

Doctor Robert B Millman, Professor of Psychiatry at Cornell Medical School, believes it does. He has coined the term Acquired Situational Narcissism to describe the destructive and outrageous behaviour of those who are constantly in the public eye. This late-acquired narcissism is characterised by almost exactly the same behaviours as the American Psychiatric Association's definition of narcissistic personality disorder (see Chapter 8). It's a phenomenon he's identified in his own celebrity patients. 'Psychoanalytic literature is full of jargon about how narcissism happens really early,' he has said, 'but I realised that given the right situation it could happen much later.'[10] He believes that narcissistic people are more likely to reach stardom than the rest of us, but once they reach the top, they often develop a full-blown narcissistic personality.

The theory is scorned by some as 'pop psychology'. But it makes sense that the power that fame and money provide literally goes to people's heads. If everyone looked at you when you went into a room, if everyone did as you asked, if everyone said you were fabulous and no one disagreed with you, wouldn't that have an effect on you? It's impossible to watch footage of Robbie Williams in front of an audience of tens of thousands of fans, every one gazing at him adoringly as they belt out the words of every one of his songs, without thinking that it has to do some funny things to his head.

Millman says that what happens to celebrities is that they get so used to people looking at them that they stop looking back at other people. That means the empathy goes, and the grandiosity grows. They begin to believe their own publicity, and think they're always right, always fabulous. That has inevitable consequences on their relationships – how can a real, giving-and-taking relationship between two people thrive on such fantasy? It also means these celebrities can be pretty poor parents – because the whole idea of 'responsibility' has become distorted for them by their life beyond parenting, where they're not expected to be responsible at all.

The lack of social norms, controls, and of people telling them how life really is, also makes these people believe they're invulnerable – superhuman almost. So they drink to excess, take drugs (these are, of course, lavish generalisations), do outrageous things like wrecking their hotel rooms, are hurtful to people and don't care about the consequences. They think there aren't any consequences – because power and money have cut them off from all such normal considerations.

This is by no means a modern phenomenon created by the celebrity age. It's something that William Shakespeare was very aware of, as demonstrated in his plays. Many of his characters are made pompous by power and money – and Shakespeare marks the point by having them constantly taunted by a Fool figure, who points out their foolishness and the way they have lost touch with reality. Think of Feste in *Twelfth Night*, who won't leave the puffed-up Malvolio alone and punctures the slightest pretension of his mistress Olivia. Or Touchstone in *As You Like It*, who goads Rosalind about her love for Orlando, and forces her to examine what she really feels. Most dramatically, there's the Fool in *King Lear*, who leads the deluded king to recognise what he is really like, and how he has imposed a misplaced vision on the world. Lear only recognises the Fool's wisdom once it is too late.

Modern-day celebrities lack that niggling voice at their shoulder, always telling them that the world they are living in is an illusion. Everyone's a 'yes man'. And once the rot has set in, it's difficult to reverse. Millman says that, as with narcissism conditioned in childhood, there's a problem persuading people that they are narcissists. You can't 'cure' them by convincing them that they're normal – because they're not, and the circumstances in which they live are bound to continue to be unusual. But he says that the actors, politicians and famous sportspeople he treats can learn to recognise a pattern in their behaviour and where it comes from, and that can help them.

The irony is, of course, that if they don't re-learn reality, then their relationships and career can all too easily fold around them. The American political psychologist Betty Glad has pointed out that once tyrants have established positions of power, their reality-testing capabilities diminish. Narcissistic fantasies that have been held in check up until they gain power are likely to become guides for action once they have achieved it, and the end result is inevitably downfall.[11]

The same can happen in celebrity-land. And once the

downfall begins, such is the hold of narcissism, even if acquired late, it is not easy to find a way back. Celebrities who lose their privileged and popular positions tend not to have a process of self-realisation as a result, recognising where their growing narcissism got out of control. Instead, anger and bitterness take hold, as they put the blame for their failure not on themselves but on other people. It's all in Billy Wilder's 1950 film *Sunset Boulevard*. When Gloria Swanson's character Norma Desmond is told: 'You used to be in silent pictures. You used to be big', she replies: 'I am big. It's the pictures that got small.'

HOW NARCISSISTIC ACHIEVERS IMPRESS US

So while some narcissistic people impress us, ensnare us even, with the appearance of success and power, a much smaller proportion will do it through actually having success and power. The charisma, the sense of self-confidence, the high ideals and aspirations are all the same and all equally mesmerising. As we saw in Chapter 3, we're probably programmed to find success and self-confidence sexually appealing, because it's a good indicator of a healthy, protective and fertile partner. And women do find successful men appealing. As the American statesman Henry Kissinger famously said: 'Power is the ultimate aphrodisiac.'

Sometimes we're drawn to people not despite their narcissistic traits but because of them. One of the more impressive things about narcissistic people is that they have an amazing ability not only to charm but to weave worlds that appeal to us. Whether those worlds are real or fantastical may depend on the particular circumstances the person finds themselves in, or their ability to get people to follow them rather than alienating them. But the line between the real and the fantastical can sometimes be a very hard one to define – for the narcissistic person as well as those around them. Several high-profile politicians, both in the UK and America, have been accused of lying about their backgrounds, and taking liberties with the truth when defending themselves against accusations. But sometimes you have to wonder whether they are actually clear about the distinction between lies and truth themselves.

As Daniel, who started our chapter, told me:

♥

There are major events that happened in my life years ago that, talking to Gilly, I realise I have completely wiped from my memory. Things I think happened this year happened years ago. Equally, she tells me there are things that I say I've done which she tells me are complete fantasy. I'm fighting the belief that I'm sane, and that it's everyone else who is crazy.

♥

It's almost as if narcissists aren't capable of lying, because their truth is a very nebulous thing in the first place. And that flexibility with the 'truth' actually can be a positive boon when it comes to convincing people you are capable of being a success in public life.

Was Napoleon a narcissist?

Napoleon Bonaparte was an expert self-publicist, creating a public image of himself that accorded with his own self-image. A magnificent portrait by the artist Jacques-Louis David[12] shows him resplendent in full ceremonial uniform, proud and determined on a rearing white horse as he embarks on a famous journey with 40,000 soldiers across the Alps to Italy in 1800. The truth was rather more prosaic. Historians believe he crossed the pass on a donkey wearing a grey greatcoat. But it was a propaganda masterpiece, and one of many portraits that reinforced a super-human image of a rather small and ordinary-looking man.

He reputedly had an astonishing self-regard – one biographer said he was 'a self-made man, and he worshipped his creator'.[13] And he had a need to create a world with his image prominent, and with others following that image devotedly.

As his influence waned, and he was imprisoned on the island of St Helena, Napoleon still created an image of himself to pass down for posterity as he dictated his memoirs. He recalled his achievements – the Civil Code, schools, roads, military victories – and portrayed himself as a saviour. And even as a prisoner he managed through his writings to create fervent followers – as high-achieving narcissists often do. 'I shall survive,' he said, 'and whenever they want to strike a lofty attitude, they will praise me.'

Notes

[1] Timothy Judge, 'Loving Yourself Abundantly: Relationship of the Narcissistic Personality to Self and Other Perceptions of Workplace Deviance, Leadership, and Task and Contextual Performance', *Journal of Applied Psychology*, vol. 91, issue 4, 2006. http://content.apa.org/journals/apl/91/4/762

[2] Manfred Kets de Vries, quoted in Diane L Coutu, 'Putting leaders on the couch', *Harvard Business Review*, January 2004.

[3] Dr Thomas Stuttaford, 'Successful leadership is all in the mind', *Times 2*, 11 September 2006.

[4] Reported in his *Guardian* obituary, by Ian Traynor, Monday 13 March 2006.

[5] Interview with Manfred Kets de Vries, 'What makes a leader great?', *Strategic Direction*, vol. 20, no. 8, 2004.

[6] Michael Maccoby, *The Productive Narcissist*, Broadway Books, New York, 2003.

[7] Marc Quinn, *Self*, 1991. Saatchi Collection, London.

[8] Tracey Emin, *My Bed*, 1998. Saatchi Collection, London.

[9] http://bigbrother.digitalspy.co.uk/article/ds11432.html

[10] Doctor Robert B Millman quoted in Stephen Sherrill, 'Acquired Situational Narcissism', *New York Times*, 9 December 2001.

[11] Betty Glad, 'Why Tyrants Go Too Far: malignant narcissism and absolute power', *Political Psychology*, vol. 23, issue 1, March 2002.

[12] Jacques-Louis David, *The First Consul crossing the Alps at the Grand-Saint-Bernard Pass*, Musée National du Château de Malmaison.

[13] Steven Englund, *Napoleon: a political life*, Harvard University Press, 2005.

8

NARCISSISM AS AN ILLNESS

Narcissistic Personality Disorder

Personality is only ripe when a man has
made the truth his own.
SOREN KIERKEGAARD, *JOURNALS*, 1843

Here's a rather shocking story that Daniel (introduced in Chapter 7) told me during our conversations:

Gilly and I had had a dog for nearly 15 years and he was largely blind and deaf. Gilly and the children were away seeing their grandma. I took the dog out for a walk. And at the end of the walk I drowned him. I could have easily taken him to the vet nearby, and had him checked over, or put down, but I didn't. Later I rationalised that it was for the best. When I saw Gilly and the children, I think I told them that the dog had died at the end of the walk. But actually, I had done it because a small but *significant part of me wanted to know what it was like to kill something sentient. It was also something to do with the drama that I could create. It was about the thrill.*

I'm not a cold-blooded psychopath. I had nightmares for a week about the dog coming out of the water to get me. Sometimes it dragged me back into the water with it.

❤

Daniel is now seeing a psychiatrist, who has given him a diagnosis of narcissistic personality disorder. NPD is a condition that, since its confirmation as a psychiatric disorder by the American Psychiatric Association in 1980, has both defined the idea of narcissistic personalities and brought the idea of narcissism into the currency of American and British culture. People like Daniel clearly have real and severe problems that, under expert assessment by psychiatrists and psychoanalysts, can be defined as narcissistic personality disorder. It is quite different from the kind of ad hoc DIY diagnoses of NPD being made by members of the public in the United States about their partners, families and friends now that NPD has become a well-known and well-publicised condition over there.

So in this chapter I want to look at what NPD is, and what it isn't; why it's a controversial diagnosis; why it's important for us all to recognise how difficult and occasionally dangerous people with genuine NPD can be; and why it's equally important for us to recognise it as an end point on the spectrum of narcissistic characteristics in human beings.

We've pointed out that some narcissism is natural – it's a primitive form of self-defence that, as we've seen in the previous chapter, can go a long way in thrusting yourself forward into the world. But NPD is not natural, and definitely not desirable, because it is a state where narcissism defines a personality to such an extent that it causes real problems for everyone who comes near. It's not common but, as Daniel's experience indicates, it can be scary, and you'll hear that it occasionally gets scarier. We have to take it seriously, because NPD can be associated with quite extreme behaviours.

As one psychiatrist told a woman whose partner had just received a diagnosis of NPD: 'Some people can hold down jobs and live well in a community and have a meaningful relationship and still have narcissistic traits. These are the sort of people one usually views as a bit cold, arrogant and aloof. Others' disorders are so severe that they are categorised as psychopaths or sociopaths. These are people who will behave in a certain way regardless of the negative, painful or dangerous effect their behaviour has on others. At the most extreme end, they will murder.'

The point at which a person with narcissistic characteristics becomes someone with narcissistic personality disorder, and the point at which someone with NPD becomes a potential killer, are difficult lines to define, even for psychiatrists. Hopefully, this chapter will at least provide some idea of why that is, and an indication of when narcissism is more than an annoyance, more even than a destructive influence on your life, and when it means you genuinely need to get some help.

NARCISSISM AS A PERSONALITY DISORDER

So let's get the facts straight first of all. NPD is defined by the psychiatrist's bible, the Diagnostic and Statistical Manual of Mental Disorders, produced by the American Psychiatric Association, as one of ten types of personality disorder.

Now a personality disorder is very different from a personality defect – which is simply a characteristic we might find personally objectionable. It's also very different from a mental illness, such as schizophrenia, which can be quite clearly diagnosed by psychiatrists, because something has obviously gone wrong with a formerly healthy brain.

'Personality disorder' has a very specific meaning among psychiatrists. It refers to deeply ingrained behaviour patterns, which are so inflexible that they tend to bring a person into repeated conflict with their social and occupational environment. There are no simple tests that can provide a clear diagnosis, and people are only judged to have a personality disorder after several psychologists and psychiatrists have spent time talking to the person concerned and their family.

According to the World Health Organization, personality disorders 'represent either extreme or significant deviations from the way the average individual or a given culture perceives, thinks, feels and particularly relates to others.' People with personality disorders, in other words, have problematic behaviour which has nothing to do with mental illness, brain disease or substance abuse – but everything to do with the way they are.

This, you will already have spotted, is immediately problematic, because it involves making assumptions about how people are normally. Many psychoanalysts are deeply uneasy about using such categorisations – because human nature cannot easily be dissected and allocated into boxes about what is normal, abnormal, acceptable, unacceptable – it is far too complex and varied for that. The difficulty is perhaps illustrated by the fact that doctors working in psychiatry estimate that up to 13 per cent of the population may be suffering from a personality disorder. Somewhere along the line there seems to be a problem with definitions if nearly one in eight of us represents a 'significant deviation' from the norm. In truth, the Royal College of Psychiatrists itself has said that current classifications are 'deficient'.

A study from the Department of Psychology at the University of Surrey demonstrated the difficulty of regarding personality disorders as independent entities that sit outside 'normality'. Belinda Jane Board and Katarina Fritzon compared traits used to define personality disorders in two groups of people – criminals/psychiatric patients with a history of psychopathy (behaviour characterised by lack of conscience or empathy), and 'normal' high-level business executives. They found that the profile of the businessmen contained 'significant' elements of personality disorder – in fact, these 'successful psychopaths' were more likely to be superficially charming, egocentric, insincere and manipulative than the unsuccessful psychopaths.[1] It illustrates, first of all, what was said in the previous chapter – that narcissistic traits can go a long way in getting people to the top. But it also demonstrates the inadequacy of personality disorder classifications, and how our judgements about whether people are disordered or not are likely to be shaded by their situation in life as much as by their innate qualities.

There's another difficulty, which makes diagnosing personality disorders very controversial, particularly in the UK. Because the diagnosis implies that a person's whole personality is flawed, how can you possibly treat it? It's simply the way people are, and you can't 'cure' them of a personality. And if that's the case, isn't it wrong to apply medical terms at all, which suggest it can be treated? The fact is that it is often the symptoms associated with personality disorders – depression, for example – that are treated, and not the disorder as a whole.

Nevertheless, various types of personality disorder have been defined, on the basis that where behaviours are consistently problematic, it is helpful at least to provide a framework for defining and understanding those problems. Each personality disorder is linked with a different set of attitudes, emotions and behaviours. While some people will have only one type, most of those who have characteristics of one personality disorder will also have characteristics associated with others.

There is no universal agreement about the different categories of personality disorder and what they constitute. In America, there are ten types of personality disorder defined by the American Psychiatric Association:

♡ paranoid personality disorder
♡ schizoid personality disorder
♡ schizotypal personality disorder
♡ borderline personality disorder (BPD)
♡ histrionic personality disorder
♡ narcissistic personality disorder
♡ antisocial personality disorder (APD)
♡ avoidant (or anxious) personality disorder
♡ dependent personality disorder
♡ obsessive-compulsive personality disorder (OCPD)

You'll see NPD is up there among all the other well-established ones. As I described in Chapter 2, it is defined by:

♡ having a grandiose sense of self-importance
♡ living in a dream world of exceptional success, beauty or love
♡ thinking of oneself as special and superior
♡ demanding praise from others
♡ feeling entitled to deference from others
♡ taking advantage of others
♡ not identifying with others' feelings

♡ envious of others, or thinking they are envious of oneself
♡ acting in an arrogant way.

Fulfilling just five of these criteria is enough, in theory, to justify a diagnosis of NPD by a psychiatrist. The American Psychiatric Association says that slightly less than one per cent of the population of the United States suffers from NPD. Similarly, borderline personality disorder, characterised by unstable and intense personal relationships and deep (sometimes suicidal) feelings of emptiness, has eight diagnostic criteria, five of which must be fulfilled. The same for antisocial behaviour disorder – which is characterised by a pervasive disregard for others and social norms.

But in Europe, psychiatrists are guided by the World Health Organization's classification of mental and behavioural disorders (ICD–10[2]), as well as the American Psychiatric Association's. And the WHO has a rather different classification of personality disorders. It consists of:

♡ paranoid personality disorder
♡ schizoid personality disorder
♡ dissocial (antisocial) personality disorder
♡ emotionally unstable (borderline) personality disorder
♡ histrionic personality disorder
♡ anankastic (obsessive-compulsive) personality disorder
♡ anxious (avoidant) personality disorder
♡ dependent personality disorder.

There's a lot of overlap between the two lists. But one notable omission in the European psychiatrists' list is narcissistic personality disorder. It's not that the World Health Organization categorisation is saying that it doesn't exist – it's just saying that it's incredibly hard to define. In fact, it specifies that narcissistic personality disorder is 'a personality disorder that fits none of the specific rubics F60.0–F60.7' (that is, the disorders listed above).

Which may help explain why narcissism, as a defining aspect of personality, is so much better known and widely publicised in the United States compared to the United Kingdom. And why, in America, narcissism is understood in a very specific sense as defining a personality disorder, whereas in the UK it is currently understood in a far more general, less condemnatory sense.

In Britain we have more of an innate suspicion of the concept of personality disorders in general, and of NPD in particular. When referred to in the UK press, NPD is invariably referred to as 'a controversial diagnosis'. In 2005, Andrew McCulloch, Chief Executive of the Mental Health Foundation, wrote a letter to the editor of the *Guardian* newspaper, asking what the point was in giving anyone the label of NPD when 'it is not clear what triggers it, it is untreatable, its "symptoms" appear to be common, albeit very exaggerated personality traits, and it overlaps with other "diagnoses".' He criticised the concept of NPD as an example of 'the dominance of a Victorian "stamp collecting" model of psychiatry'. In other words: such diagnoses are a mark of a determination to impose medical ideas on characteristics of the mind and human nature, which cannot sustain them. The important thing, he said, was to develop psychological techniques to help people with such extreme personality traits.

The letter puts its finger on the great problem with making something like NPD into a defined and accepted 'condition'. NPD is a very useful concept, because it helps us identify something important and destructive in some human beings. But it is much more problematic when used as a label to tie to individuals, because the label is notoriously difficult to apply, and doesn't actually help those it is applied to. That's why we've got to be careful in using the term.

There is another perspective on this. Thousands, if not millions, of people around the world have had their lives adversely affected by people – often their partners – who clearly have dramatically narcissistic personalities. For them, the need to have a label to characterise the personality of those who have caused their suffering becomes a necessity. Not only can it help them feel less of a victim, and less to blame for some of the dreadful things that have happened, but it can also provide a means by which to isolate the people who caused them such suffering from the normality of everyday life, and in so doing protect others from any dangers they present. It can be used as a strong statement that these people are simply not normal.

Psychiatrists have an angle on this too. Because there comes a point where narcissism, and the personality disorders associated with it, becomes so far from anything compatible with human society that it has to be (to use a word much loved of sociologists) 'pathologised' – in other words, treated as an illness, even if it cannot be cured.

So the label of NPD, for all its difficulties, is necessary for both psychiatrists and those affected by people with strongly narcissistic personalities. The measure of someone with NPD is how demoralising, disturbing and dangerous their behaviour is. A person has more than narcissistic traits, and has a narcissistic personality disorder, when they consistently cause more problems than they solve. What's more, their world view will be so ingrained that they will be totally unable to see themselves as the cause of such problems, and their ways of coping with the situation will inevitably make things worse. You can tell a person with NPD because of the vortex of deepening chaos that engulfs them and the people around them.

We heard above that some psychiatrists believe that some people with narcissistic personality disorder are so disordered that they can be categorised as psychopaths or sociopaths. Another way of looking at it is this. Psychopathy and sociopathy are becoming slightly outdated terms in psychiatric circles – many psychiatrists use the concept of personality disorders instead. In particular, the term antisocial personality disorder is used to describe those people for whom the term 'psychopath' used to be used – those who demonstrate lack of remorse, irritability, deceitfulness. It is in this crossover between NPD and other personality disorders like antisocial personality disorder that the real dangers may lie. In people who have both narcissistic and antisocial personalities, the lack of feeling for others, the lack of conscience and the lack of inhibition can become overwhelming. They believe they are above the rules of normal society. The lines of distinction are hard to define, but understanding this may help us begin to understand the point where disordered personalities become dangerous.

PERSONALITY DISORDERS AND CRIME

In July 2004, 19-year-old Brian Blackwell, a public schoolboy, battered his father to death with a claw hammer, stabbed his mother 30 times, then went on holiday to the United States with his girlfriend – paid for on his father's credit card. He spent £2,200 on a three-night stay in the Presidential Suite of the Plaza Hotel, New York, then travelled to San Francisco, Miami and Barbados, before returning home to Merseyside. All the while, he acted as if everything was normal, picking up his A-level results on his return, and celebrating with teachers and friends that his hard work had brought him four straight As. It was only in September, when neighbours noted a bad smell coming from the Blackwells' bungalow, that his crime was discovered.

Brian Blackwell was sentenced to life imprisonment for the murders a year later. The five psychiatrists who assessed him were unanimous in their verdict: he had narcissistic personality disorder.

Schoolfriends nicknamed him 'The Brains'. His parents, Sydney, 72, and Jacqueline, 61, from Melling, Merseyside, hoped he would become a surgeon. He was due to take up a place studying Medicine at Nottingham University. But for all the outside appearances of normality, Brian Blackwell was not a normal teenager.

He was expert at weaving lies – perhaps because, like many full-blown narcissists, he believed them himself. And it all had its root, somewhere, in truth. Blackwell was a good tennis player – captain of his school team, and under-eighteens north-west champion in 2003. But he told his girlfriend Amal Saba that so high was his ranking that he had been given £70,000 by Nike in a sponsorship deal – he even showed her forged contract documents. And when Amal could find no confirmation on the internet, he convinced her that his ranking wasn't listed yet. 'I thought there's no way anyone could make up such a detailed lie and never hesitate when questioned,' she has been quoted as saying subsequently.[3]

Having convinced his girlfriend that he had the money, Blackwell took her to view a £59,000 Mercedes sports car, bought her expensive-looking jewellery (actually cheap silver), and offered her £80,000 a year to be his personal secretary (her first salary cheque bounced because Blackwell was overdrawn). Needing money to prop up his fabricated idea of himself, he took £9,000 from an investment account his parents had set up to pay for his university, convincing the bank that his father had died and he needed to buy a car to support his career as a tennis player. He bought Amal a £6,500 Ford Ka with the money.

The illusion was, of course, unsustainable. His parents discovered what he had done, and demanded that he ask Amal for the car back. They told friends they would never again trust him with money, but Blackwell tried to find other sources of income, applying for loans and credit cards on the basis of his fictional life as a professional tennis player. His parents blocked his attempts.

But Blackwell had promised Amal a holiday. On 24 July he booked flights to America using his father's credit card. The next day he killed his parents, packed his bags, and left with Saba for their £30,000 trip.

On his return more than two weeks later, Blackwell didn't go back to the family bungalow. After all, his father's body still lay undiscovered in the armchair where he had been killed, and his mother's in the bathroom. He stayed with his girlfriend's parents, claiming he was locked out of the house until his parents returned from holiday. The bodies were only discovered weeks later, and finally Blackwell's fantasy could be sustained no longer.

During police interviews, Blackwell said he had been hanging pictures in his bedroom and had a hammer. 'His mother and father had been out having an evening meal and had returned home,' said Detective Inspector Geoff Williams of Merseyside Police. 'After a few drinks there was an argument between Brian and his father. It resulted in a fracas between them in the living room.'

The prosecuting lawyer in his case said there was nothing to indicate that Blackwell had premeditated the killings. He told the court that sufferers of narcissistic personality disorder typically fly into a rage if their fantasy world is threatened. Blackwell, he said, was 'a highly abnormal young man'.

Blackwell's neighbours, questioned by the press after he was found guilty, couldn't agree whether he was normal or abnormal. Neighbour Margaret Smith, 73, said he was a 'lovely, quiet lad'. And 75-year-old Tommy Sheldon said he was a 'very clever lad' who studied hard. But several neighbours have pointed out that Blackwell was dominated and cosseted by his mother – who bought his clothes, and bathed him until the age of 17. The pressure on him to succeed, and fulfil his parents' aspirations for them, seems to have been strong. 'His mother was inclined to be strict with him,' said Tommy Sheldon. 'He was not allowed to play with other children,' said Margaret Smith.[4]

What are we to make of this? Well, first of all, one can conclude that all the characteristics of narcissistic personality disorder are there. There's the blurring between fantasy and reality, the lack of understanding of others, the grandiose romantic gestures, the anger when the illusion begins to disintegrate, even the indications of strict and possibly controlling parents.

What is clearly disturbing is that this man's narcissistic tendencies seem to have contributed to murder. For those who have contact with people with narcissistic characteristics, it raises the obvious question: how can you tell whether a narcissist might be dangerous? The warnings were certainly there that Brian Blackwell was a compulsive liar who built a fantasy world. But could anyone have predicted, even if they had surmised all this, that he would have lashed out in such a violent way? Is it possible to predict whether narcissistic personalities are dangerous?

The answers to these questions are annoyingly indefinite. But they may be reassuring too. First, we have to acknowledge the fact that the vast majority of people with narcissistic personality disorder (who constitute around just one per cent of the population) are not dangerous. For the very few who are dangerous, it's probably not their narcissistic traits by themselves that make them potentially violent, but a blend of uncompromising personality disorders that bring a lack of conscience and responsibility for actions. For the fact is that personality disorders (and personalities) are rarely neatly self-contained – if a person fulfils the diagnostic criteria of one type of personality disorder, he or she often fulfils the criteria of at least one other. Many of the men we have discussed in this book have traits that would certainly tick several boxes on both the narcissistic and the borderline personality disorder scales.

The psychoanalyst and psychiatrist Jeremy Holmes put it very nicely when I talked to him: 'Most people with NPD don't murder their parents,' he said. 'They may leave a trail of miserable people and failed relationships behind them, but they don't murder. One way of thinking about this is that the more personality disorders you have, the more disordered you are. It's rare to see someone as dangerous as Blackwell. That's not to say that some murderers aren't narcissists – but it may be antisocial personality disorder and not narcissism that's the key to that.'

In fact, in Britain, the whole idea that people with personality disorders are dangerous per se has become a very politically contentious issue. In 2001, Michael Stone was given three life sentences for killing Lin Russell and her six-year-old daughter Megan, and for the attempted murder of Lin Russell's other daughter, Josie. The three were attacked with a hammer on a country lane in Chillenden, Kent, in July 1996. Stone had already received a diagnosis of severe antisocial personality disorder, but because his personality rather than a mental illness was the root of his problem, the authorities had not been able to detain him under mental-health laws. In response to the case, the government proposed new legislation that would allow people with personality disorders to be detained, even if their condition were untreatable (as it usually is with personality disorders).

There was outrage from some mental-health groups. They pointed out that although the proposal was to put only people with severe personality disorders in detention centres – the probation service estimated that there were 4,000 of them – it could be very difficult to distinguish severe cases from moderate and mild cases. Mental-health charities such as Mind were flooded with calls from people with personality disorders, worried they were about to be locked up. The plan was eventually dropped as the government realised the implications of effectively imprisoning large groups of people who had never committed a crime. In late 2006, however, it resurrected the plan, trying to ensure that compulsory treatment is given even to those with psychiatric problems that cannot easily be cured.

The assumption that people who have been categorised as having personality disorders are killers is indeed a very dangerous one. It belies the true picture, that most people with personality disorders are intensely problematic but not violent. And it fails to take into account the fact that even psychiatrists believe the way that personality disorders are defined and applied is flawed. They can never be certain of their 'diagnosis' – unlike diagnosing heart failure or cancer, you cannot diagnose a type of personality. If you took a brain scan of a person, there is no narcissism lobe you can examine for signs of enlargement. Pinning down a personality is like dissecting a cobweb.

Which brings us back to the idea of narcissism itself, and why, when we wonder whether people we know have narcissistic personalities, we need to remember that narcissism is a way of understanding people, not an illness. Our interest in narcissistic personality disorder should not mislead us into believing that we can diagnose people with narcissism, and load all the problems we've had with them into the file marked NPD. Rather, the idea of narcissism allows us to identify, hold and characterise some of the defining aspects of personality. NPD helps us define a type of personality where self-centredness, arrogance, grandiosity and an inability to appreciate the emotional lives of others have been carried to an extreme. We should not assume that this makes all people with those extreme qualities alike, or believe they have identical propensities for love, violence, anger, cooking, throwing darts or anything else.

So if we accept that one per cent of the population has narcissistic personality disorder, how many of this group are at the psychopathic extreme of NPD, where conscience and normal rules go by the board? It's impossible to say. But it is a tiny fraction of that one per cent.

It may sometimes suit us to characterise a group at the extreme end of human behaviour or experience as villains or monsters, but the unpalatable and difficult truth is that for all their subjective repellence, they are always human.

Notes

[1] Belinda Jane Board and Katarina Fritzon, *Crime and Law*, vol. 11, no. 1, March 2005.

[2] This is an abbreviation used for the International Statistical Classification of Disease and Related Health Problems (10th revision) – it is a means of doctors, nurses and other health professionals recording health problems. It is published by the World Health Organization, available online at http://www.who.int/classifications/apps/icd/icd10online/

[3] 'An unspeakable crime', *The Sunday Times Magazine*, 9 October 2005.

[4] 'Killer Blackwell's fantasy life', BBC News, 29 June 2005. http://news.bbc.co.uk/1/hi/england/merseyside/4634401.stm

9

THE HOLLOW MEN

What it's like to be a narcissist

> *A man is a God in ruins.*
> RALPH WALDO EMERSON, *NATURE*, 1836

What's it like to be inside the head of people with strong narcissistic traits? What do they really feel about themselves and why they do what they do? This chapter is necessarily brief because we know very little about how it feels to be a narcissist. That's because most narcissists find it so hard to face up to their inner self, are so bolstered in self-belief by their long-held defence mechanisms, that they wouldn't even contemplate describing themselves as a narcissist, and would never describe how it felt. They are blind to their own behaviour – it's simply what is normal to them, and getting them to talk about narcissism in anything but an abstract way is like asking a deaf person what they can't hear.

We can, however, get glimpses. First, there are now chat

rooms on the internet where some men and women who acknowledge they are narcissists are revealing their feelings. The anonymity of the internet has provided them with a means to explore issues that have perhaps niggled at the edges of their minds for a long time, egged on by others like them who are recounting their experiences. These people talk about their confusion, their desperation at the fact that they cannot maintain relationships, and their guilt at the destruction they are causing.

And then we have Daniel, first discussed in Chapter 7. He's a 36-year-old man who's being forced to face up to his narcissism, because last year psychiatrists gave him a diagnosis of narcissistic personality disorder. As a result of that he talked to me honestly and bravely about how it felt to be him.

Daniel is obviously not your average narcissistic male. He's high-spectrum narcissism, with his behaviour having created significant problems for himself and those around him. But unlike your average low- to middle-level-spectrum narcissist, he's prepared to talk about his problems and his complex emotions. People like Daniel, who have been challenged about their behaviour because it is causing significant problems, are forced by psychiatrists to look at themselves more objectively. So they provide an insight into the thought processes, motivations, and inner emptiness of lesser, as well as greater, narcissists.

Perhaps what these accounts demonstrate most of all is that narcissists shouldn't be written off simply as villains. Difficult as they are, they exemplify the way most people, in one way or another, build protective mechanisms to conceal their inner inadequacies.

Daniel's story

Around eight years ago, Daniel was diagnosed as having a borderline personality disorder – something he now says he has no recollection of. But when he was forced by his wife Gilly to face up to the fact that there was something very wrong with him (something we'll hear more about in the next chapter) he visited a private psychiatrist, and the whole of his life history started taking on a different perspective.

❤

I'm absolutely terrified now I'm seeing a psychiatrist. I was trying to explain to Gilly the other day how it felt having to face the fact that I had a personality disorder. And it's like for most of my life I have been driving a car down the wrong side of the carriageway, and only in the past twelve months have I been shaken into recognising for the first time that I'm going the wrong way. It's so terribly difficult to stop the car and go with the flow.

It's a good analogy because it starts to explain why the roller-coaster ride is so attractive. Driving on the wrong side of the road can be exciting and gives you a sense of uniqueness. It makes you very much the centre of attention. Now I've got into this very tricky situation where going with the flow seems excruciatingly dull. It's like living life in the grey.

My career is in tatters. And I have no friends. Actually, I have one friend who I have known since I was fourteen, who I grew up with, and he's a friend despite how I am.

Until I started to change in the last twelve months, the inevitable feedback when I met people was that I was disliked. It's something that gradually got fed back to me by my wife – that somehow I gave out a vibe of something between antagonism and depression and was seen at best as haughty and at worse as dismissive, arrogant, cocky and destructive. I seem to make everybody I meet feel deeply uncomfortable. If you imagine it being like that wherever you go, it leads to a very lonely life.

The common image of a narcissist is someone who is in love with themselves, but it's really not that simple. No part of me gets any pleasure from being disliked. I want to walk into a room and for people not to say 'Who is that odious shit with Gilly?' Not only do I seem aggressive to people, but throughout my life I have shown no real interest in them. Yet I still feel I deserve their attention. That's the central contradiction. People talk about narcissism in terms of self-love, but it's simply not like that.

I want everyone and everything to behave as I wish, and that makes life very difficult. It's tiring being the world's policeman. I edit life according to my wishes. Looking back, I realise that's what I've done with timescales and memories – I change things to suit my story. And I try and push people into behaving in a certain way, the way I want. That's exhausting.

The other misconception is that the life of a narcissist is charmed – that somehow, because of their tremendous self-belief and latent ambition, enormous success follows. But it's not like that either. At the core of what I feel is a profound emptiness. And the pursuit of thrills, and the roller-coaster life, the sexual exploits, and the binge eating are all trying to fill a gap which is always there. I've tried taking flying lessons and driving racing cars but nothing ever fills the hole. And the trouble is that you want your wife to fill it for you, and that's terribly destructive. Because there's no way she can do it, but you're somehow forcing her to. The sense of emptiness is profound and omnipresent but strangely not there all the time.

Trying to face up to the fact that the whole of my life up until now has been based on something so empty and worthless is hard. It's like ... well, imagine you're in the dark, you can't see, you have no torch, you have no idea where you are, where you came from, and no idea what road to take. You have no map in terms of a past to tell you where you are and where you should be heading. It translates into an absence of self-awareness and self-belief and purpose.

For most of the time I've been married I've been a disastrous husband. I've always looked for my wife to satisfy every need that I've had, whatever it is, which is impossible. And I've set her standards that she couldn't possibly meet. Yet I've routinely criticised her. I've undermined and mocked every success she has achieved because I'm jealous of it. I've tried to belittle her and reduce her circle of friends. It's been a stream of building her up to knock her down. And I'm beginning to realise now that it's about projection – by saying she is shit at something, I'm actually saying that about myself.

I vacillate between believing I'm magnificent and believing

I'm profoundly ugly and I look frequently for validation from other people that I look okay. If I don't get it, I get into a cycle of depression and start binge eating. In terms of sexuality, and this is offered to you in all modesty, when I want to, and when the circumstances are right, and if I find the right individual, I can be as compelling to a certain kind of woman as a lamp is to a moth. I don't know how or why, and there is some kind of subliminal radar that allows me to pick on the right individual. And I can make that person lose all control to satisfy me.

I did it with a work colleague. What I had in mind to do to her was drive her crazy, because I had initially treated her with total disdain, and when I turned the lamp on it made her feel as if she were the only person in the world. Another woman actually left her husband and pursued me for some time. She ended up going to a psychiatrist because of her strength of feeling for me. Nothing happened with her, but I just had this effect on her, because I wanted to. That feeling of power is addictive.

💛

It's an impressive account, isn't it? Daniel builds a beautiful story, struggling for self-awareness, lost, eloquent. What's also fascinating is that talking to Daniel, and reading what he said, it's hard to know what to take at face value. Remember, he is a narcissist, and what he says shows many of the hallmarks of a narcissist – his charm and allure shine through, but so does an awareness of the drama of it all. Is there something self-pitying here? Or is he just being painfully honest? Is his account of his past and his present self-glorifying, and possibly fantastical? It's hard to tell.

Let's try to pull out some of the central strands of how it feels to be a narcissist, as illustrated by Daniel and by some of the male and female narcissists now contributing to narcissism discussion groups on the web. Remember that any person who contributes to such discussions has at least partially acknowledged that they are a narcissist – and that means they're not representative of the vast world of people with narcissistic tendencies out there. But what they say reflects not only the group of severe-end narcissists who are being forced to face themselves. It also reflects some of the characteristics of less severe narcissists who have never been completely blind to their inner failings.

Ashamed

For most of the time I've been married I've been a disastrous husband.

Some men and women who have narcissistic personalities have moments of self-awareness. They may repress them, but some have an abiding inner voice quietly telling them that the way they are behaving is wrong. When you bear in mind that narcissists tend to be the way they are because of an in-built lack of self-worth, conditioned in their early childhood, it's not surprising that the inner message that they are behaving despicably is an extra-hard one to face up to. Someone like Daniel has moments of hating his appearance, because of his inner lack of self-esteem, and then everything else accumulates on top of that.

It's described as shame or self-loathing by narcissists. They say they were made to feel ashamed when they were infants and children – possibly by their inability to conform to their parents' wishes – and have felt inwardly shameful about themselves ever since.

Here's what a man who set up his own website to face up to his narcissistic characteristics has to say about this:

♥

'I don't know the origins of my behaviour, meaning I don't know whether it was nature or nurture that made me the man-beast that I am, but I can tell you the effects. First, there's the self-hate and stress. By this I mean I was always cleaning up after myself and hating myself for whatever I just did. Most often, it was treading water to keep my head above a lie or actions that pre-cipitated a lie. Second is the stress on those around me, like my parents or my beleaguered wife or the family reputation. There was also an effect on peripheral lives.

♥

Fearful
I'm absolutely terrified now I'm seeing a psychiatrist.
Those narcissists who do have an inkling of self-awareness – and as we'll see in the next chapter, it's something that usually has to be forced upon them – can start to feel very frightened. The fear can take two forms. Some less severe narcissists, or those who are facing up to their behaviour, have some awareness of

the effects of their actions on others around them. If they have families, they fear for their safety. More common, however, is fear about how they can cope. Once they begin to see the barriers and artificial world they have created around themselves, the world can look very scary indeed.

Here's one male contributor to an online narcissists' discussion group whose fears lie in the effect on his family: 'I have never been physically abusive – my wife and kids are very special. That is part of the reason that I want them to go – to protect them ...'

Others are expressing fear of facing up to their real selves and the real world:

❤

My biggest problem with my narcissistic tendencies is that I'm too scared to try/do/be anything in case I fail, and make myself aware of just how crap I really am.

If I don't put any real effort into it, then I'll know that I could have done it if I really tried. Because I'm so brilliant, and so much more intelligent and gifted than everyone else ... But then if I actually tried, I might fail (gasp) and I just couldn't cope with that. I'm terrified of both failure and success. It's a maddening paradox.

❤

It's quite characteristic of some narcissists, for all their apparent self-confidence and will to change the world in their image, to actually end up doing nothing. Stuck in a rut of non-productivity, because they are afraid (usually subconsciously) of the failure that will destroy their idea of themselves. These are the non-productive narcissists, the polar opposite of the productive narcissists we saw in Chapter 7.

The creator of the website again sums up nicely how it feels once you realise you are not 'normal'. For him, the fear is also mixed with anger about himself:

❤

Now, I won't lie. I want to be honest from the beginning. I am in therapy because I am the most emotionally barren person I know. It's so bad that I suspect I must be a genetic mutant of some sort. I am absolutely unmoved by anyone's suffering, including my own. I always believed in the cruelty of blind fate: that everyone always gets what they deserve anyway, including me. So I won't stretch the truth and say that what I feel about my past actions is remorse. I'll say that anger and fear – the only two emotions I can truly identify when I feel them – are ever-present when I recall my life thus far. I'm angry about things I've done. I fear my callous ability to go through with some of the worst things. I fear my wife coming to her senses and leaving me. I fear that I can never be emotionally normal, and that fear makes me angry, somehow.

❤

Heartless

At the core of what I feel is a profound emptiness.

Many narcissists talk about being 'emotionally barren' or feeling 'emptiness'. It worries them that something very important is missing. It also worries some of them that the opposite of feeling emotionally attached is very much present – they get a positive kick out of being unpleasant to people. They worry that it actually makes them feel in control, alive. All in all, it adds up to narcissists feeling heartless.

Here's a female narcissist, trying to trace that feeling back to her own upbringing:

♥

With relationships, there's a fear of intimacy/loving because I think I've learned to equate loving someone with being abused/controlled. I am a chameleon. I can be whatever they want me to be, and OMG I always get the 'we're soul mates', 'matched in heaven' blah blah blah … pass the bucket! After a while they get attached to me, want to see me all the time, wanting to be with me … and I start seeing them as pathetic and weak, so I devalue them and look down upon them. Sometimes I get the urge to just play games with them. I think that might be a subconscious way for me to get back at those that hurt me when I loved them (my mother). For me, loving equals control, so when someone loves me, they want to control me.

♥

A male writer describes a strange compulsion to be wicked to others:

♥

I never realised it before, but I want to be cruel sometimes. That sounds sick, I know, but I have always idealised characters in movies and books who have no conscience, and can just pull the trigger. I had 25 girlfriends in the three last years of school. I hunted, literally, the most difficult prey, chameleoned into their ideal, and then took what I wanted.

♥

And another correspondent describes how tantalising and painful it is to see others feeling things deeply, but to be unable to feel similarly himself. This, he believes, may have something to do with narcissists' natural envy.

♥

I make jokes, I laugh, I cry. But the emotions that cause these physical reactions are so shallow and so fleeting that seeing someone moved to true joy or sadness leaves me nothing but bewildered. As if they were trying to explain advanced mathematics in Icelandic. Other people's emotions, in fact, disconcert and confuse me so deeply that I often find myself hating people who show emotions around me. It's envy, pure and simple. I think, 'Why should this jerk be able to weep with joy when something happens while I stand here like a burnt-out light bulb?'

I feel like I am emotionally one million years behind the human race. I am self-preservational and libidinous, and my emotions are barely there, save the aforementioned fear and anger, those reptilian emotions that even crocodiles have. The scariest part is that I'm smart enough to know that my feelings are retarded and [I] cannot will them into existence. Imagine having a giant, painful, throbbing boil that you cannot reach or see, but that you know is there. That's my emotional life.

♥

Lonely

No part of me gets any pleasure from being disliked.

Daniel talks about how fed up he is of having no friends. It's not true that all narcissists are friendless, but many do talk of being isolated, and comment on the way that people seem to drift away from them. One writes: 'I have no friends except my wife, but she is leaving in four days to go home. She's taking our kids with her.'

Exhausted

I want everyone and everything to behave as I wish, and that makes life very difficult.

As Daniel says, it can be tiring being a narcissist. You've got to spend a lot of mental (and sometimes physical) energy making sure that you assert yourself on the world, and ensuring the world conforms to your vision. Narcissists often talk in terms of feeding off others, and others providing their 'narcissistic supply'. It's as if they have a permanently depleted tank that needs refilling with other people's emotions and energy.

Here's a female narcissist talking about her relationships, and how they alternately feed her and then exhaust her – setting up a constant cycle of demand and supply.

♥

In the honeymoon stage at the beginning of a relationship, I am mirroring back at them exactly what it is they are looking for in me. This produces the 'Wow, we are like soul mates or something!' response in the other person, which is what I am looking for. They think I'm special and amazing, and they feed me their energy. But I can't keep that kind of thing up for longer than a few weeks or months. Because it drains me. Then I'm tired. They already think I'm great. I've become the centre of their world – now they want me to feed them my energy and attention.

♥

Trapped

That feeling of power is addictive.

Narcissists, like their partners, often feel trapped. But unlike their lovers, wives and partners, narcissists are trapped of their own volition. Some know they are stuck in a rut of antisocial behaviour and attitudes – and have a vague awareness they should change. Perhaps that is why so many conduct rapid image changes of clothes or hair. But changing deep down is virtually impossible for them. To them, the way they are is normality, and changing a normal life for the life that others lead is like jumping out of an aeroplane. There may be a vague desire to change nagging away, but real will can be impossible to find. It feels safer to stay the way you are. As one website correspondent puts it:

❤️

I want to disappear for a while, grow my hair long, study psychology or philosophy, and re-create my life. I know 're-creating' is not a good idea, but I like creating lives. My wife thinks I am going to see a psychologist, stay on my anti-depressants (I will), and spend some time with our priest, get better, and then go back to Europe and live with her and the kids. Here's the problem – I don't want to change. I like me. Yes, I have just lost my beautiful wife and kids and my job – but I have no intention of seeking change in the immediate future. This, if nothing else, confirms to me that I have narcissistic personality disorder.'

❤️

So how hard can it be for narcissists to be brought out of that comfort zone of normality, to try to address their real personalities? That is what we will look at in the next chapter.

10
CONFRONTING NARCISSISM

Getting help

*Question: How many therapists does it
take to change a light bulb?
Answer: Just one, but the light bulb
really has to want to change.*

ANON

So let's say you're rapidly coming to the conclusion that someone in your life is a narcissist, or that a narcissist is ruining your life. What do you do now? Get out of the relationship while you can and run for the hills? Or try to change things – try to develop coping mechanisms that will make life more bearable, try to confront your partner with their narcissism and encourage them to change?

Well, first of all, there's a lot of support for the 'run for the hills' school of thought. It's very much in evidence in American sources of advice. Of the many web-based discussion groups that have recently arisen where 'victims' of narcissism air their tribulations and describe the chaos narcissists are wreaking on their lives, there is one called 'N magnets anonymous'.

A man I spoke to recently applied to join the group. He was concerned that his wife was a narcissist, and wanted to get some advice about what his best course of action was. He was rejected. This is the response he got from the group moderators:

♥

Our site really doesn't deal with helping one to live with a narcissist. Our only 'advice' is to run, and to run far and fast and to not have any contact with them. Those at our site who are trying to 'make it work' with a narcissist are spinning their wheels.

Since you seem to want to stay with your wife, we really aren't the right place for you. If you are ever ready to join us, you'll know. If your wife is truly a narcissist, then you will always be in a 'no win' situation.

♥

The reply was written with the best of intentions, but left the man – who had invested a lot in his marriage and children over nine years – feeling bereft. The email was written from the standpoint that you can never change a narcissist. To an extent, this is true. It's a counselling truism that one partner cannot change the other – all they can do is look at themselves, and how they are contributing to problems. And we've seen in the previous chapters, narcissism is not an 'illness' but an attribute of personality, and therefore not something that you can 'cure' as such because it's part of you.

And yes, it is true that in the case of extreme narcissistic personalities, getting out and far away is usually the safest thing to do. People with narcissistic personality disorder will always be incredibly hard to live with, and are sometimes a danger to the emotional and physical health of others. The chances of them ever transforming their intrinsic characteristics, forged since birth, is virtually zero. As one woman I spoke to said: 'You can't change someone's personality. It's like trying to cure liking the colour blue.'

But the discussion-forum moderator failed to acknowledge two things. First, that even people who have strong narcissistic characteristics can be confronted with their behaviour. Sometimes, this can give rise to at least a transient desire to change that can result in dialogue. That dialogue can lead to further conversations, sometimes with psychoanalysts and psychiatrists, that can help them to understand and avoid certain behaviour patterns. It can lead to treatment for some of the associated by-products of a narcissistic personality, such as depression and aggression, which can make living with them far worse.

This is by no means a given, and the more extreme narcissistic cases are unlikely to last the course – psychiatrists say they often dismiss counselling as stupid after a couple of sessions because they can sense it threatening their sense of self. It's well-recognised that one of the defining characteristics of people with narcissistic personality disorder is that they see themselves as superior to their therapists, and regard all their problems as nothing to do with their own traits. It's other people's fault. But some people – as we shall see – can stick with treatment to some degree, and feel a benefit that also benefits others. It's not that they are 'cured', but that they cope better by understanding better.

This links to the second point unacknowledged by the group moderator. If a man believes his wife is a narcissist, it doesn't necessarily mean she has narcissistic personality disorder, or even a narcissistic personality. It could mean she has some narcissistic traits – ticking the boxes in our first questionnaire in Chapter 2, for example, but not in the second one. With a bit of open discussion between partners, and maybe some intervention by an expert relationships counsellor, there might be a considerable improvement in the relationship.

It's not easy, especially when the narcissism is extreme. And it doesn't always work. This chapter concentrates on what can actually be done to help someone with narcissistic traits. We'll see first of all how challenging it can be to confront extreme narcissism – both for the narcissists and their partners. Then we'll move on to how to confront narcissistic traits that are less extreme.

HOW NARCISSISTS FEEL CONFRONTING THEIR PERSONALITY

Can someone with a narcissistic personality be cured? According to Gilly, whose husband Daniel has been diagnosed with narcissistic personality disorder, the answer is clear. 'One of the things I'll never have is closure. That's the thing about personality disorders. You can't cure them.' But she's living with the conviction that Daniel can be helped. After all, she has a personal stake in it. After eleven years of marriage, she decided finally that something had to be done, and made Daniel face up to things. This is how Daniel describes what happened:

There was a pivotal point where I had to begin to face the question of whether I had a personality disorder. It was when Gilly, in total exasperation, virtually pushed my face in front of the computer and made me read the diagnostic criteria for various mental disorders and made me check them off, one by one. I think, somehow, she just caught me at the right point. There was a realisation that my work was in tatters, I was being horrible to the children, I had no friends, and perhaps Gilly was going to leave me. I'd become aware of my total dependency on Gilly, and felt very lonely and pathetic. Maybe there was a bit of maturity kicking in too, who knows? But I know that before that point, with my face against

the computer screen, I could never have been at fault. But then the possibility did enter my mind, and I did agree to go to a psychiatrist, privately. I didn't want to continue being disliked.

❤

So for the past year now, Daniel has been seeing a psychiatrist. Neither Gilly nor Daniel are sure whether it's going to do any good long-term, and it's certainly hard for both of them. Daniel is very conscious of the fact that he's suddenly meant to be living without any of the protective strategies he's always relied on. The psychiatrist has prescribed some medications to try to help him depend on the old strategies less.

❤

The thing I'm wrestling with at the moment is all the defence mechanisms that my personality disorder makes me rely on. So I have medications for depression, mood changes and anger. But you can't medicate narcissism. And there are some things that I'm failing at. When Gilly and I talk about the things that need to change, I say to her that I feel like a pencil drawing that's gradually being rubbed out. It's hard to know what will be left when all the defence mechanisms are gone, and I'm floating in the grey, and don't know where I am.

❤

Gilly is pleased that something, finally, is changing, but she too has doubts. 'The drugs do make him behave much better and he's nicer to me when he's taking them. But what does that mean? When it's a personality disorder, is it still him? Is it real?'

These are common themes. Here's another account from a man, Paul, reluctantly trying to face up to the fact that he needs to change. His thoughts very much echo Daniel's:

❤

I am afraid of what will happen if I do resolve my problems. I won't have any more excuses. My future will all be down to me, and I'm afraid of what that might involve. It will probably mean I have to start doing things like everyone else – get a job, behave responsibly, get people to like me, and create a social life. I will have to be humble and conform so I can fit in. And among all those other billions of people living normal lives, I fear I will become lost. I may be bettered by people who are stronger than me, and will have to accept that I no longer have the divine right to rule, and will just be another guy.

❤

Here's another man, describing that vital leap that has to be made – to really want to be helped.

❤

If you're going to allow yourself to face the fact that all your life you've been avoiding something really bad about yourself, it's got to be the most important thing in your life to you. You have to want to confront it so much. I'd be very surprised if anyone ever reaches a place like that without going through periods when they think they're never going to achieve anything, and might as well give up. That's certainly true for me.

❤

Such personal testimony is eloquent and fascinating. Narcissists, when they do tell their story, are extremely good at it – because they project and dramatise themselves. They communicate just how hard it can be to face up to their nature, and go and get some help.

But Paul, Daniel and Gilly may take some consolation from this account, from a man who has taken the leap, has been consulting a therapist for months, and has felt real benefits:

❤

Therapy helps you become aware that you do have real feelings inside you. When people first said to me that my anger was fuelled by something very deep inside me, I felt very threatened. But then, talking it over with the therapist, I came to know myself much better, and I recognised what they had been saying was true – that I actually got angry when people told me something very true that I just refused to acknowledge. This eventually became a conscious awareness – so that I could recognise what I was doing, when I was doing it. The whole process was incredibly difficult. I remember the first few times I met the therapist, we just talked about life in general, sport and politics, but at the end of that he suggested moving on a bit to look at what my problems were, and that was enough to send me running for a few months. I did that a few times, but I kept coming back, and I'm glad I did.

❤

Perhaps most heartening of all is this short anecdote, from a man who posted his experience on the internet. He swears he used to be completely unable to feel pain, either physical or emotional:

❤

One day my therapist asked me what I do when I feel pain. I responded that I don't feel pain. He found that quite amusing. It took me quite a while to understand that I had been feeling pain all of my life, and what I had been doing with those emotions was avoiding them, hiding them behind some incredible inner walls. The process of allowing yourself to experience what you've spent a lifetime avoiding is painful almost beyond words, but it is also incredibly rewarding.

❤

HOW TO HELP SOMEONE
CONFRONT THEIR NARCISSISM

It is a hard business for partners of people with strong narcissistic traits to try to convince them of their problems, or demonstrate the destructive effect they are having on the lives and happiness of others. People who have relationships with narcissists are often sucked up into a world not of their choosing, where the rules are different, and it's difficult to dictate or guide anything. If the laws of gravity don't apply, it's hard to keep your feet on the ground. We'll see in the next chapter how sometimes the very nature of the relationship, and the nature of both partners, not just the narcissist, can get in the way of effectively addressing anything.

One psychiatrist informed me that the best thing to do if you want to make a narcissist face up to pressing issues was to ignore them, and if that didn't work to leave them. That was the only approach, he said, because they found it so hard to blame themselves for anything, or face the need for change. He's not alone in that belief. But these people are generally referring to very extreme narcissists, and there are many other psychiatrists and therapists who point out that some strategies do maximise your chances of helping a narcissist embark on some creative self-reflection. They are, in fact, some of the same strategies that may help you also live a more constructive life with a narcissist, which will be dealt with a little more in the next chapter.

The experience of relationship therapists is that the couples who tend to do well – the couples where narcissism is confronted, and where a solution (whether splitting or staying together) is sorted out – are those who talk. It's not rocket science, and it's the secret of most good relationships and problem-solving. But it's a means of constantly reflecting back on the other person what you're feeling, and impressing on them the implications of certain things that have happened in your lives. Having a joint social life and some constant friends and relatives in your life is also a good thing, for similar reasons. It provides a safe and non-threatening environment where there is constant and sometimes subtle feedback about what's right, what's wrong, and how people are feeling.

This can be easier said than done. It suggests a normality of everyday life that in cases of extreme narcissism can be difficult to create. Nevertheless, for people who live with lower-spectrum narcissists, it's an environment that will gently challenge, but not threaten. This is very important.

'As a partner, it's about reflecting a consistent response,' says Dr Quazi Haque, a forensic consultant psychiatrist at the Priory's Farmfield Hospital, who has treated many people with extremely narcissistic personalities. 'It's a matter of being very clear about what's right and what's wrong, but in the process not rejecting your partner, because that's very threatening to them. Be clear that something has to change, but you aren't going to abandon them. That can be very difficult because these conversations often happen after a row. But if you do have a row, always try to follow it up with support.'

So here's the rub. If you decide that leaving your narcissistic partner is the best option – and it is a legitimate option – that's one thing. But if you really want to try to move things forward, to try to improve things between you, you're going to have to confront your partner with their behaviour. But there's a difference between confronting and being confrontational. It's a question of presenting them with the facts, but in a non-threatening manner. That means not threatening them with being kicked out if they don't change, or using other emotional blackmail (though that might only seem fair given the amount it's been tried on you). The fact is that people with strongly narcissistic traits fear abandonment. It's all to do with the reason they probably became narcissistic in the first place – they're people who have often been abandoned emotionally by previous people in their lives. So if, for the moment at least, you've decided you're not going to leave them, then you have to make it clear to *them* that you're not. If they think they're going to be abandoned again, they're going to feel threatened, and that will simply make them resort to all those age-old defence mechanisms that make their behaviour so intolerable, and communication so difficult.

Confronting them does, however, mean doing something to make them think, and this may be an ongoing process. There may be no revelatory moment, no key encounter, as there was for Gilly and Daniel. But over a period of days, weeks or most probably months, an environment can be created where it is more likely that a person with narcissistic traits will be able to stare their true characteristics more fully in the face.

Here's a summary of what you can do:

♡ Avoid isolation.
♡ Try to surround yourselves with genuine friends and relations.

♡ State your case strongly, but reassure the person you are not going to abandon them.

♡ Create situations where you have to talk – if you've constantly got the television on, or are making yourselves busy, then talking openly is much less likely.

♡ Try to convey how you feel things – and how the things that your partner does affect you.

♡ Try to avoid doing this in the context of an argument.

♡ Be firm and consistent about behaviour you find wrong or hurtful.

♡ Try to encourage others in your close social circle to draw a similar line, and tell your partner when they find behaviour hurtful or unacceptable.

♡ Being emotional is fine, but try not to get into situations where you say things you don't mean.

♡ Encourage the person to ask questions about their own behaviour and personality traits.

THERAPY FOR NARCISSISTIC PERSONALITIES

In terms of the 'official' treatment narcissistic personalities receive from psychoanalysts or psychiatrists, this tends to be an extension of the sorts of strategies mentioned above. Therapists, however, have an objectivity unencumbered by all the other baggage and grind of day-to-day relationships, and this can bring extra benefits.

Let's assume that something has happened, some crisis, some culmination of a long-term process of discovery, which has made someone with narcissistic traits agree to go to see a psychiatrist. Most likely it will be a professional at a private clinic. In severe cases of destructive behaviour, which might suggest narcissistic personality disorder, an NHS referral would be possible in theory. But consulting a family GP about this can be embarrassing, especially if there's the threat of stigma and getting sucked into the NHS mental-health system. So private or charitable help is usually the most realistic option (see contacts at the end of the next chapter).

There are four basic rungs on the treatment ladder:

♡ establishing trust
♡ addressing the source of dysfunctional thoughts and behaviour
♡ identifying the 'symptoms'
♡ developing a new language, and new strategies.

In all therapy, it's important for the person to feel a sense of engagement and trust with the person treating them. But it's especially important for narcissists and people with personality disorders, because they unconsciously fear investing trust in anyone. With trust comes the implicit danger of abandonment. Sometimes psychiatrists and psychoanalysts spend weeks or months simply talking about things on a completely non-threatening basis to build some sense of belonging and engagement. As one psychoanalyst told me:

❤

I've had a lot of narcissistic clients, but it's often the case that unless there's an awful lot going wrong in their lives, they won't come and get therapy. During therapy, they tend to respond very badly to anything remotely critical. They have very grandiose images of themselves, and get very defensive. There are some areas where you find it very hard to go. Narcissistic people only want to hear the good news, and once things appear to get better they'll walk out, and you have a job getting them back again. When you start to address anything problematic, they have a tendency to just say something like 'bloody useless therapists'!

❤

As trust develops, a therapist might explore the origins of dysfunctional patterns of thought and behaviour – invariably found in past relationships, and most significantly in relationships with parents and caregivers. The fears of abandonment, and where they arose, need to be addressed. When these difficult areas are broached, then so can be their consequences.

'In many of these disorders,' says consultant psychiatrist Dr Haque, 'the individual grows up having poorly integrated ideas of themselves – especially in relation to their identity, sense of culture, beliefs and impulses. Some have a limited self-awareness about their emotional lives, and a stark lack of emotional language to express how they feel.'

So part of the treatment is to begin to learn an emotional language, identifying certain feelings and how they are associated with dysfunctional behaviours. 'It can be useful to think of these behaviours as symptoms, which can be more predominant in certain situations and with certain stresses. It's quite common, for example, for people to feel more threatened if they become stressed, and if they feel threatened they may revert to basic primitive responses such as aggression and heightened suspiciousness.'[1]

The next stage is to try to identify some of the trigger points for dysfunctional behaviour, and how to avoid them. It's about being able to predict which sorts of situations are going to be most provocative or stressful for a narcissistic person, and developing strategies for either avoiding these or replacing the self-defensive strategies with something less destructive. Psychiatrists talk about developing 'alternative scripts'.

For example, a man who had a stepfather who regularly criticised him as a child, and hit him when he had done badly at school or otherwise 'failed', may have grown up constructing defence mechanisms around himself which swing into action every time he feels stressed, or threatened with the possibility of failure. Every time he comes across anyone who may be doing things 'better' than him, including his partner, he might go into a pattern of withdrawal, drinking heavily, and then expectedly lashing out. This is a pattern that might not be obvious to him, or his partner, but may become apparent when some situations and the feelings they induce are reflected back at him. As he develops an emotional language, this process will become easier. If that pattern of hiding away is identified, it might help both the person and those around them identify the first signs of it – and develop new 'scripts' that don't automatically lead to violence.

This isn't about changing your personality. But it is about changing patterns of behaviour that lead to unhappiness, and can end up causing an escalation of destructive feelings and situations. It is something that partners themselves can help instigate, and if psychiatrists are consulted they should involve the partner in this process.

HOW MEDICINES MIGHT HELP

You can't treat narcissism with drugs. But people who have trouble recognising their own emotions and have a very fractured sense of self will often have associated problems as a result – they may be depressed, for example. A psychiatrist or GP might prescribe antidepressant medication to at least control this particularly corrosive side effect.

In some people with narcissistic personality disorder, psychiatrists also use medicines to help control some of the more extreme manifestations of the person's personality – aggression, say (for which drugs called anti-psychotics are sometimes prescribed), or extremely impulsive behaviour (for which antidepressants called SSRIs are used). This is what Gilly earlier described feeling so uneasy about – worried that the medications were making her husband actually less like her husband, even though they compensated for some of his most extreme behaviour. But psychiatrists do think they are useful as a means of ameliorating many 'symptoms', and trying to break any vicious circles of destructive behaviour.

In America, a doctor called Leland Heller has cut across the psychiatric mainstream by saying that personality disorders are actually treatable in their own right. He says that conditions like borderline personality disorder, which is commonly found in association with narcissistic personality disorder, is actually a 'medical disorder masquerading as an emotional one', and therefore prescribes medicines as a cure. Use, for example, of the antidepressant drug Prozac, he says, is 'a platform that allows people to recover'. He says he has treated over 3,000 'border-lines', but his work, based around the belief that personality disorders have a physical cause, remains controversial.

HOW SUCCESSFULLY CAN NARCISSISM BE CONFRONTED?

'Treatment' can only be applied to complaints that potentially improve as a result. Since you can't cure a personality, some would say that attempts to confront narcissists are bound to fail. But there are narcissists and narcissists, and though the problems of constructively changing someone with extreme narcissistic tendencies are self-evident, it is self-defeating to write off all attempts to help those with less extreme traits.

As Dr Quazi Haque says:

❤

It all depends on the kind of disorder, and the individual's ability to develop trust. Narcissists tend to look for external validation, for messages that they are great from the outside. The degree of how 'outward' they are in this search can be indicative of how well they respond to treatment. The extremely egotistical people who struggle to accept rules and have little sense of boundaries or the perspectives of others can be extremely difficult to treat. They reject treatment because theirs is a world of impulses and pleasure seeking. But for others, it's different. It all takes time, and you have to maintain the idea of a trusting relationship, and let them talk and project and express the need for validation. But you can gradually wean them off certain patterns of behaviour.

❤

ACCESSING HELP

The sub-heading of this chapter is 'Getting help', and it is impossible to over-emphasise how important getting support is if narcissism is genuinely adversely affecting your life. Narcissism is not a problem unless it's causing problems. If it's causing you problems, then get advice from people who know something about what to do. In the United States there are dozens of self-help books about narcissism, dictating to readers what they should do about certain types of personalities in certain circumstances. But human personalities and human relationships are too complex to deal with in tick-box solutions. If you're in trouble, talk to an expert. There is a list of people and organisations that can help you at the end of the next chapter – a chapter that addresses perhaps the most difficult subject of all: what you can do to extricate yourself from the destructive power of narcissism, and perhaps save your relationship at the same time.

Notes
[1] Quotations from phone interviews conducted with Dr Haque in 2006.

11

IT'S ALL
ABOUT YOU

Confronting your future

*Whoever loves becomes humble. Those who love have,
so to speak, pawned a part of their narcissism.*
SIGMUND FREUD

Why, exactly, can it be so hard for a partner of a narcissist to act in the face of their partner's difficult, sometimes disastrous, behaviour and attitudes? Whether it's a case of getting up and getting out, or talking openly, or simply asking for help, there can seem to be insurmountable obstacles.

Here's Gilly talking about the sequence of events leading up to her confronting Daniel with the fact that he really needed help:

♥

I became aware of how things had become, and that something had to be done, both gradually and suddenly. I had been living in a situation where things were extreme and scary for a long time. Daniel likes to isolate me and keep me away from friends and I was finding it difficult so I was making an effort to do more stuff and see my friends. That had made me ask what's normal and abnormal in my life. At the time, Daniel was incredibly depressed and desperate. He did nothing all day long, but I was having to work full time and look after the children. He would speak to the children in a way that was hurtful and upsetting to them. Nothing was as it should be. And all those things added up. And the more I saw my friends, and the more I was aware of what they thought, the more I thought there must be something wrong.

You'll remember that Gilly eventually sat Daniel down in front of a computer screen to examine for himself all the characteristics of someone with narcissistic personality disorder, and to ask himself how much it tied in with his own behaviour. But that was a full six months after she'd typed 'lack of empathy' into Google, and became convinced of what was wrong with him. Why didn't she talk to him sooner?

There was an element of fear, but that wasn't everything. I'd been going to see a therapist myself for the past year, and each time I saw her she asked me 'Have you had enough yet?' And eventually, I came to that point. I had to rub Daniel's face into all the characteristics of personality disorder that he had.

But Gilly still feels almost paralysed. It's partly the situation that Daniel has put her in, and the psychological effect he's had on her. But it's also something about her. She simply won't leave Daniel.

♥

I feel as if the life I want is just out of reach. It's a bit like Dorothy when she was in Oz. On an intellectual level, I know I could change my life as easily as she got back to Kansas, but emotionally it feels impossible. It's as if I live in a different place to all my friends and the leap is so huge that I might fall and never recover.

Plus, therapy never really worked for me, because my therapist simply wanted me to find the strength to leave the relationship and ended up getting frustrated with me. She tried all sorts of tactics, including telling me that I'm setting my daughters a very bad example of how a relationship should be. I understand that totally – she's probably right, but it's just so incredibly hard to put into practice.

♥

If you're in a relationship with someone with narcissistic traits, you'll have read this book while recognising some of the ways your life has been made difficult by your partner. You'll have read about all the ways that a narcissistic person can make you feel – powerless, demeaned, belittled. And guilty. You'll probably feel – even if you're trying to repress it – that in some way you've contributed to the whole mess you're in, and the bad behaviour of your partner.

Okay, so here comes the hard bit. You probably have.

Now before we go any further, let's make clear that this has nothing to do with fault or blame. You'd be wrong to feel guilty about the difficulties encountered in your relationship. But you may be right to think you're playing your part in what's going on, and how you're feeling about the whole situation. Because the fact is, if you're in a relationship with a narcissist, and it's proving problematic, you can't isolate those problems from yourself. You've got to look at you too.

There are several reasons for this. First, we fall in love with people for a reason. It's not just about some pure concept of love that each of us pulls down from the ether when we clap eyes on 'the one'. Our lovers fulfil needs in us. Try to think what it was that attracted you to your partner in the first place? Are the things that you found attractive and the things that are incredibly disruptive to your life and happiness now different sides of the same coin? Could it be that what you now see as selfishness and lack of empathy was actually an attractive trait of confidence and self-sufficiency when you fell in love?

It's been pointed out by more than one commentator, and it's something we drew attention to in Chapter 3, that people who themselves are the products of narcissistic parents seem to be particularly susceptible to the charm of narcissists. It's not always clear-cut. But it's certainly true that we are all needy in some ways, and we choose lovers who fulfil those needs, who make us feel better about ourselves.

In the case of Gilly, she confessed to me that she thought she was 'co-dependent'. This is a term that has only recently been bandied around in the field of relationships and psychotherapy, but it has an interesting and specific meaning. It means the tendency to put others' needs before your own, and to accommodate others to such a degree that you tend to discount or ignore your own feelings, desires and basic needs. Co-dependents' self-esteem depends largely on how well they please or take care of others. It's not difficult to see why co-dependent types and narcissistic types might be drawn together.

This isn't to suggest that people who enter relationships with narcissists are 'damaged'. It simply means that, as with all of us, their past relationships have conditioned certain needs and vulnerabilities. It's part of what it is to be a human being.

All couples bounce off each other. Our patterns of thought and behaviour are continually influenced by those around us, and in particular by those we live with or have relationships with. Because partners are important to us, because we spend a lot of time with them, what they say and do can have a deep impact on us emotionally even if we don't consciously recognise it. As we saw in the previous chapter, our vulnerabilities and insecurities can be triggered by everyday events that in the course of our relationships can go unnoticed and unanalysed. We all spark off good things and bad things in each other, and couples invariably have to look at how they interact together to get to the root of the emotional problems of one, or the other, or both. We're involved, whether we like it or not.

Finally, it's about you because you have feelings about the whole situation. You have to address them and look after yourself – you can't look at the situation as something you have to 'solve' for everyone else. You have to try to resolve it for yourself, and that requires looking at yourself: how you feel, what you're like, and what you want. You're not going anywhere without that. As one woman who had recently finished a relationship with a narcissistic man said to me: 'There was a point where I just told myself to snap out of it. Women can be their own worst enemy, and you do sometimes have to ask whether you just need to decide what needs to be done, and do it.'

Finally, looking at yourself as well as your partner is the only way to approach things constructively – at least, it is if you've made the decision that you want to stay together. You can't make a partner change, but you can make changes in yourself. In doing so, you can break some of the cycles of thinking and behaviour that cause conflict. So if you really want to make a go of it, you've got to look to yourself, and how you're contributing.

So that's why it's all about you. In the rest of this chapter we'll take some of those realities a little further by providing advice on how to analyse your own situation as a couple, and some practical strategies on how you can progress. It involves looking at yourself, looking at how the two of you might be interacting together, asking some difficult questions about what changes can be made, and deciding on a way forward.

YOUR PERSONALITY

So let's start off by looking at your own personality a bit. What characteristics might you have that are contributing to the way you're feeling about your partner? This is particularly important to consider if you're distressed about the situation. You may be able to determine how you can try to change your own reactions to certain situations.

Try thinking about the following:

☐ Do you feel responsible for other people's happiness?
If you do, it may be making the whole situation far worse for you. Narcissists will find people like this much easier to manipulate into feeling guilty and beholden.

☐ Are you a caring sort of person?
Some people have an automatic instinct to look after others, even when they can look after themselves. The problem with this is that it can encourage people to become dependent on you, rather than independent of you. Again, this can present problems if you have a partner with narcissistic traits, because it leaves you open to becoming trapped.

☐ Do you overestimate how much you should be able to control life?

People who do this inevitably feel guilty – a lot. There's only so much you can control in life at the best of times, but if you're in a relationship with an impulsive and unpredictable person it can be virtually impossible. Being like this can make you feel a failure – and that sort of low self-esteem will be made worse by someone who constantly needs to make themselves feel superior.

☐ Do you always have high expectations?

This is connected with the question above. Expecting a lot from yourself and from others has many positive sides – at work, for example. But being a perfectionist can also lead you to seeing everything that doesn't reach your high standards in a very negative light. That includes you. If you're very self-critical anyway, you'll feel it very deeply when your partner starts picking holes in your behaviour or attainments.

☐ Do you tend to feel others are better than you?

This can cause extra problems for people who have relationships with narcissists – it can make you more likely to do things you wouldn't normally do, especially if it is a way of avoiding demeaning comments from your partner, which are likely to make you feel even more worthless.

☐ Are you frightened of relationships ending?

Like narcissists, those who get into relationships with them can fear abandonment too – for many different reasons. If you think that your very survival is dependent on maintaining the relationship, that can throw up many difficult issues which may be affecting your judgement.

☐ Do you have a history of difficult relationships?

This is perhaps the most complex question of all. Our relationships with parents, siblings, friends, relatives and work colleagues shape our lives. From the moment we are born, they help define who we are and how we feel about things. If in the past we've felt disappointed or betrayed in a relationship, then we'll inevitably feel cautious or even suspicious about future ones. This is understandable, and happens to all of us. But it can give rise to particular types of emotional hypersensitivity, insecurity or lack of trust, which inevitably affect how we relate to people. Here are some of the common life experiences that counsellors and therapists encounter in their work with clients which seem to be influential here:

♡ Having parents who expect you to know what they want and take responsibility for their wellbeing.

♡ Having parents who are emotionally detached – sometimes simply because of absence.

♡ Feeling isolated or lonely as a child.

♡ A chaotic family life where you never knew what to expect of people or situations.

♡ Feeling rejected or devalued – your parents or a partner seem to think you're not good enough.

♡ Feeling that someone – a parent, former lover – has betrayed your trust.

♡ Feeling frequently blamed for things you didn't have control over.

All of these experiences from upbringing and past relationships (some have been suggested by counsellor and psychotherapist Nina W Brown in her book *Loving the Self-Absorbed: how to create a more satisfying relationship with a narcissistic partner*[1]) might provoke certain feelings, worries and behaviours. In turn they may affect how you feel about your current relationship, because it's very easy to impose the expectations conditioned by a past relationship onto a present one. They may influence the way you're reacting in certain situations, the things that stress you out, the things you say and the vulnerabilities you display. Perhaps most importantly of all, they may explain why you can't act – why you find it impossible to leave, or address the situation.

Look back at the case studies, and ask whether the women who have told their stories in this book show signs that some of these influences – high expectations, a caring nature, difficult past relationships – might be relevant. Might they be influencing the way they feel about their partner, and their decision-making (or lack of it)? It's not at all surprising if so. Many exemplify quite admirable empathetic traits often found in women.

If you understand what you are doing, it can be the first step towards seeing your current relationship more objectively and finding a way forward. But remember this process of self-analysis isn't always simple – it requires an objectivity that is hard to achieve by yourself. It can also easily turn into a process of self-blame, which is the last thing you want. That's why these things are often best addressed with a personal counsellor, a marriage counsellor, or a therapist.

WORKING OUT WHAT TO DO

Getting professional advice and support is often the best policy if you have problems in a relationship. But people often don't know when a breaking point has arrived. When have things got bad enough to get help? When, for that matter, have things got bad enough that you should leave rather than stay? How do you begin to assess your situation?

It's never an easy process in any relationship, let alone relationships where your sense of reality and self-esteem can be warped. But the following advice should provide you with a framework on which to base some important decisions.

Assess your situation objectively
If you feel you can't see things objectively any more because you're so sucked up into your situation, make an effort to get out a bit and take part in some activities that give you distance, a sense of self-worth, and a perspective beyond life with your

partner. Get a life. If the person you're in a relationship with reacts badly to this, try to assess why that is, and use it as a starting point to determine whether you can address your problems together. Discuss it with him or her if you can.

Try to look coolly at the past and present, and realistically assess how the future looks in the face of it. If you're finding it hard to see things objectively, ask how you'd feel if a daughter or sister were in this situation. This can be especially useful in assessing whether there's any real risk of physical abuse, and worrying behaviours like serial infidelity, sadism, violent anger and deceit. Of course, if there are children in the household, then there will be an extra reason for playing safe and removing yourself.

Surround yourself with support

This applies not just to you, but to your partner too. Having friends and relations around you provides a sense of security, continuity, and a safe environment where issues can sometimes be addressed. If nothing else, people outside the relationship can reflect back your behaviour as individuals and as a couple, to provide some kind of feedback on what they find acceptable, and what is not. Some of this feedback may be just subtle social signals. But sometimes your friends might tell you some home truths too. Try to listen to them, and don't automatically assume that everyone else doesn't understand. What they say may not always be an accurate reflection, but it can provide a valuable perspective with which to examine your own thoughts and assumptions.

Assess exactly how narcissistic the person is

The checklists in Chapter 2 will help. But it's important here to make a genuine assessment of the person you're having a relationship with. Are they someone who you can work with, or someone who it's virtually impossible to work with because they're a full-blown narcissistic personality?

What you're looking for really is an indicator of where they sit on the narcissistic spectrum. As Dr Haque indicated in the previous chapter, the narcissists who are the most 'treatable' – in other words, the narcissists who are capable of change – are those who aren't entirely dependent on the outside world for their sense of validation. Many people with narcissistic traits are still capable of being giving, being sympathetic and trying to understand. When it comes to trying to make a relationship work, these people are very different from extremely egotistical people whose actions seem unaffected by the wishes or feelings of other people. So look for signs of sympathy and good intentions. You don't have to have a personality disorder to find change hard – all of us find changing ingrained habits and patterns of behaviour difficult. Sometimes it's a matter of sheer complacency or laziness. And remember that we all have a vein of narcissism in us that is occasionally bound to rise to the surface.

On the other hand, remember that true narcissists are very good at appealing to our softer emotions, swaying us with moments of sensitivity and vulnerability, which provide us with an excuse for saying: 'Oh, he's quite normal really.' What you need to look out for are consistent signs of a caring attitude. If they are sporadic and mixed up with abominable behaviour, this could be the sign of a true narcissist trying to get you back on his or her side, rather than any genuine good intentions.

Assess if there are grounds for believing you can work it out together

This is the key one, because ultimately it determines whether you get professional help, and whether you stay or leave. According to Paula Hall, a relationships psychotherapist and counsellor with relationships advice charity Relate, there are three key areas to consider:

- [ ] Does the other person accept the need for change?
- [ ] Do they want to change?
- [ ] Do they have the capacity to change?

If the answer to the first question is no, and has been consistently no even when the person has been confronted with their unacceptable behaviour and the effect it's having on you, then there may be no need to even look at the other questions. If the person wants to change, that's certainly the prompt to get some professional help. But if, after that, you honestly believe they don't have the capacity to change, there may be nowhere to go but the door. You have to assess what, realistically, is the possibility of change. If you think it's zero, and you're desperate and unhappy, it may be time to get out – no matter how much you have previously invested in your relationship or your family.

'Some of this process,' says Paula Hall, 'may involve asking the questions: "Does the person have a vested interest in staying the same, and if so, what is it? Why has the person not changed up to now?"'

Work out if you need professional help

Working out when you need professional help isn't actually that difficult – because lots of couples with even seemingly minor problems have benefited from seeing a relationships counsellor. Relate recommends that a good time to consider expert outside help is when you seem to be going round in circles as a couple, repeating the same arguments, getting in the same difficult situations, and not having any new ideas about how to approach the problem. 'But don't wait until you've exhausted all the options if everything is meanwhile falling apart,' says Paula Hall. It's certainly worthwhile getting expert advice if you're feeling desperate or vulnerable, or if the other person's patterns of difficult behaviour seem to be escalating, or if you're both becoming increasingly distrustful of each other.

Remember that this isn't as daunting as it might sound. Seeing a relationships counsellor is the sensible thing to do if one or both partners is simply troubled in the relationship – there doesn't have to be World War III breaking out. And getting expert help doesn't indicate that your relationship is on the rocks – on the contrary, it indicates you're prepared to invest in working things out.

Relationships counselling is sometimes a first step, and sometimes it's enough. Some individuals achieve quite significant personal growth in just six sessions of relationship education. Often, it's the beginning of a longer process involving further work by the couple, and sometimes additional therapy or counselling either individually or together. Strongly narcissistic people will need intensive psychotherapy if there's ever going to be an improvement in the relationship. But couples counselling is always an extremely useful entry point into accessing help and embarking on a bit of self-analysis for people who would never accept that they might need psychiatric or psychotherapeutic help themselves. Even if they can't see a problem in their personality, they might be persuaded to see that there is a problem in the relationship. And that can be a vital foothold in moving things forward.

Unfortunately, there is no state system for helping couples through relationship problems in the UK. If you want to access help, you're going to have to pay for it – but Relate does offer subsidised services that may be cheaper than private couples-counsellors. If you do choose to go for private counsellors for relationships advice, do try to make sure they are trained in couples counselling.

Should I stay or should I go?

Leaving is always an option. If you leave, you will survive, and heal, and those you leave behind will probably be okay too. Don't necessarily view leaving as the last resort – especially if the situation is in any way dangerous. It may be what you should have done years ago. The perspective of friends and professionals will help. Don't convince yourself that everyone else is wrong apart from you – that, after all, is what narcissists do.

Work out what you would do if you stay

It might be something you do before getting expert help, or afterwards, but at some stage, if you've made the decision that you're staying with your partner, you're going to have to work out a strategy for addressing how to make things better.

In the previous chapter, we heard how one of the key areas to work on is to try to identify the situations that seem to exacerbate the narcissistic person's troublesome behaviour. Are there some events that they seem to find particularly stressful? Is the stress associated with some of the things you do? Are there strategies you can work out, hopefully together (because this isn't a matter of you constantly making compromises for the sake of peace and quiet), for making those situations less provocative to the people concerned? If, for example, the person tends to resort to alcohol if feeling neglected – which makes them more angry and unpredictable – can you acknowledge that together, and work on finding another less destructive outlet? Are there certain social situations that actually you both find quite stressful, and would rather do without?

Your strategy will have to involve confronting the issues with your partner. Be clear that something has to change, but communicate that you still want to be with them – if you do.

According to Paula Hall, one strategy that sometimes works with people who aren't showing much empathy is to try treating them the way they treat you. It has to be done for a limited period, and you have to explain to them why you're doing it, and why it isn't a sign that you hate them. Saying to someone 'See how it feels' can be quite a hurtful and threatening thing if done the wrong way, and can make people erect impenetrable defences. But if you can put 'See how it feels' into action in a non-confrontational way, it can hold up a mirror to behaviour, and be more illuminating than a simple accusation. Emphasising that it's not about what's right and wrong, but about what's healthy for the relationship, may help.

Another way of making your partner view their behaviour more judgementally is to ask them how they would feel if a child behaved in that way. Would they tell them off, and want to try to prevent them doing it again? Sometimes people can wean themselves off behaviour patterns once they see that they wouldn't like them in anyone else. In narcissistic personalities it's a much more difficult prospect than for most people. But it can be done.

If you've tried to do these things before with no success, and haven't yet got outside help, part of your strategy must be to get expert advice.

PEOPLE WHO CAN HELP YOU

Relationships advice and counselling

Relate

Provides couples with counselling about their immediate problems, either face-to-face, by email or over the phone. There is normally a charge. For more details see www.relate.org.uk or phone 0845 456 1310.

Tavistock Centre for Couples Relationships

Provides couples counselling with a more psychoanalytical approach than Relate, examining some of the formative issues that have made people the way they are. For more details see www.tccr.org.uk or phone 020 8938 2353.

2as1

A national organisation for the black community in Britain, providing a first port of call for anyone needing marriage and relationship support. For more details see www.2as1.net or phone 0700 222 2700.

The Institute of Family Therapy

A family therapy organisation offering services for families and couples facing a wide range of relationship difficulties. For more details see www.instituteoffamilytherapy.org.uk or phone 020 731 9150.

Individual counselling and psychotherapy

The British Association for Counselling and Psychotherapy

Can put you in touch with qualified psychotherapists and counsellors. For more details see www.bacp.co.uk or phone 0870 443 5252.

UK Council for Psychotherapy

Provides access to the Council's register of psychotherapists. For more details see www.psychotherapy.org.uk or phone 020 7014 9955.

British Psychoanalytic Council

An organisation for therapists who specialise in psychoanalytic psychotherapy, which aims for deep-seated change in personality and emotional development. Provides access to its register of practitioners. For more details see www.bcp.org.uk or phone 020 7267 3626.

British Psychological Society

Can help you find counselling psychologists who assist people in managing difficult relationships and life events. For more details see www.bps.org.uk or phone 0116 254 9568.

Psychiatric help

Royal College of Psychiatrists

Provides information about mental illness, and advice on finding NHS or private psychiatric help. For more details see www.rcpsych.ac.uk or phone 020 7235 2351.

MIND

The mental-health charity with a local network which specialises in providing individual support. For more details see www.mind.org.uk or phone 0845 766 0163.

The Priory

Priory Healthcare is a private source of psychiatric help, with centres around the country. For more details see www.prioryhealthcare.com or phone 01372 860 400.

Notes

[1] Nina W Brown, *Loving the Self-Absorbed: how to create a more satisfying relationship with a narcissistic partner*, New Harbinger Publications Inc., Oakland CA, 2003.

BIBLIOGRAPHY

Carter, Dr Les, *Enough About You, Let's Talk About Me: How to Recognize & Manage the Narcissists in Your Life*, Jossey-Bass, San Francisco, 2005.

Hotchkiss, Sandy, *Why is it Always About You? The Seven Deadly Sins of Narcissism*, Free Press, New York, 2003.

Lasch, Christopher, *The Culture of Narcissism: American Life in an Age of Diminishing Expectations*, W W Norton & Company, New York, 1979.

Lowen, Alexander, *Narcissism: Denial of the True Self*, Simon & Schuster, New York, 1985.

Maccoby, Michael, *The Productive Narcissist: The Promise and Peril of Visionary Leadership*, Broadway Books, New York, 2003.

Solomon, Marion F, *Narcissism and Intimacy: Love and Marriage in an Age of Confusion*, W W Norton & Co, New York, 1989.

Acknowledgements

This book is dedicated to the people who took the leap of faith to talk openly to me about how it feels to be a narcissist or in a relationship with a narcissist. For some of them it was a potentially dangerous, as well as emotionally demanding step, and the book wouldn't have happened without them.

I'd also like to thank the following for the advice and considerable expertise they offered to me: Paula Hall, Quazi Haque, Jeremy Holmes, Michael Knight, Andrew G Marshall and Bel Mooney.